Praise f
bOObs: A Guide

"We thought our Boob I(
is a real fountain of brea
we are smarter, more
And our girls rock.

—Samantha Schoech & Lisa Taggart,
editors of *The Bigger the Better, the Tighter the Sweater*

"Give me an A! Give me a B! Give me a DD! Squires brings
us a book that is equal parts celebration, affirmation, and
information. Illuminating and entertaining, bOObs is
all about getting in touch with your girls."

—Tania Katan, author of *My One-Night Stand with Cancer*

"A breast-friend's guide to owning boobs, and a testimony
to their influence on our culture at large."

—Rebecca Apsan, author of *The Lingerie Handbook*

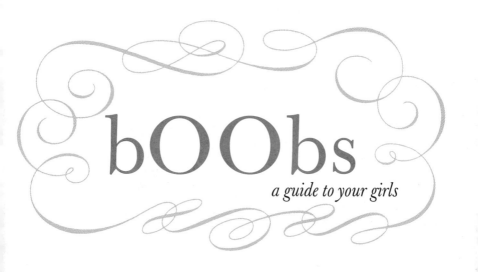

bOObs

a guide to your girls

ELISABETH SQUIRES

SEAL

bOObs
A Guide to Your Girls

Copyright © 2007 Elisabeth Squires

Published by
Seal Press
A Member of the Perseus Books Group
1400 65th Street, Suite 250
Emeryville, CA 94608

Library of Congress Cataloging-in-Publication Data

Squires, Elisabeth.
Boobs : a guide to your girls / Elisabeth Squires.
p. cm.
Includes bibliographical references.
ISBN-13: 978-1-58005-207-8
ISBN-10: 1-58005-207-X
1. Breast—Care and hygiene—Popular works. 2. Brassieres—Health aspects—Popular works.
3. Breast—Examination—Popular works. 4. Breast—Diseases—Popular works. I. Title.

RG492.S69 2007
618.1'9—dc22
2007016664

Cover design by Gerilyn Attebery
Book design by Kate Basart/Union Pageworks
Printed in the United States of America
Distributed by Publishers Group West

The information contained in this book is for general interest only. The author is not a
physician, and no information found here should be used for medical purposes—diagnostically,
therapeutically, or as a substitute for the advice provided by your own medical professional.

For My Mother

Contents

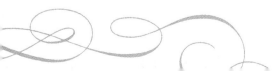

Introduction

Do women *really* know their breasts? If so, why do

- 80 percent wear the wrong size bra;[1]
- 89 percent overestimate their risk of breast cancer;[2] yet
- only four out of ten perform monthly breast self-exams?[3]

GET ABREAST

If we can't dress them, we're scared of them, and we won't touch them, what else don't we know? Let's face it—boobs are everywhere. And everyone seems more focused on how they look rather than how they work. Anchored as they are to us, we may assume our breasts are a known quantity. They are, after all, *just* another body part, right?

Our relationship to our breasts seems a bit different than to other areas of our bodies. We may rarely touch our bosoms unless looking for something wrong. We might allow others to handle them—lovers, doctors, or a nursing child. We may show them off in some strapless or other low-cut gown for that special occasion. We may hide them away if they draw too much attention—or feel inadequate if they don't. Even a woman who is satisfied with her breasts may still wonder if they'll be altered by time, circumstance, or (more likely) gravity. Will they support us or let us down?

If we like our breasts, we project a positive and confident image to the world. If we're dissatisfied in some way—pesky bra riding up on our backs, shoulder straps too loose or too tight, wires digging into our skin—it can make us cranky and miserable. And the world sees us that way, too. We can choose to celebrate our unique qualities (and buy a better-fitting bra while we're at it), or think that our breasts' distinct nature makes us flawed and deficient. It's really all in how we look at our own breasts.

But we don't think about our breasts every day. There are some days we completely ignore them, until something happens to make them the focus of attention. When we go for a run or a swim, we become aware that they're fairly gelatinous in nature. They won't stop jiggling, or they bolt out of place without warning. Or maybe our swimsuit has stiff, built-in cups that feel false. When it's "that time of month," they're swollen and sore, and none of our bras seem to fit. When we buy a cute, trendy top we're anxious to wear, we go home and find we don't have the right bra to complement our outfit. Then we shake our heads and wish we'd inherited some other size or type or that we were built like a friend or a colleague (whose boobs *are* perfect . . . even if we've never actually seen them).

Many young women are confused when their breasts first appear on their bodies and wonder whether their size or rate of growth is normal. Some of these anxieties can stay with us for a lifetime. How can we make our daughters feel proud and confident about their bodies? Young girl or mature woman, we're seldom comfortable talking with each other about our breasts. Is there something our lovers need to know? Do the things they do or say about our breasts change our view of ourselves? Even if accustomed to the never-ending search for the most comfortable bra for our body type, we're still faced with outfitting ever-shifting cup sizes during pregnancy, nursing, and beyond. Our breasts are altered by diet, exercise, and plastic surgery, too. We may even turn to pills and potions to improve our busts.

With pink ribbons plastered everywhere, breast cancer is on the minds of many women. We may want more information about breast diseases and how to know when our breasts are healthy. We might wonder when we should have our first mammogram and what we can expect during this procedure. Someone we know might have been recently diagnosed with breast cancer, and we want to know how we can help during this difficult time. What causes breast cancer, and why haven't we found a cure? Which charities should we support? Does

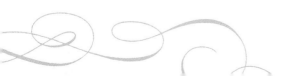

diet and exercise affect our own personal risk, or are there environmental factors we can avoid?

What about the safety of silicone implants? Many women's breasts are of an unusual size and shape; some of us may want information on cosmetic surgery, its risks and rewards. If we undergo hormone replacement therapy, our breasts will change in other ways. We may just want to know where to buy one *great* bra for our aging breasts.

Can women live happily ever after with breasts as they reflect their changing lives? We find articles in various magazines on different topics, but where is the one place we can turn to for comprehensive advice and information? *bOObs* provides answers to the many questions we have about breasts. It's an owner's guide to our very breast friends.

THE BIRTH OF *bOObs*

My inspiration for this book came sometime after my forty-seventh birthday, when I made a decision to celebrate my upcoming fiftieth by getting my body in the best possible physical shape. I kicked butt every day at the gym for a year, taking up jogging for the first time ever and lifting weights. With my three "babies" nearly full grown, I had the time to be more consistent about exercise, and I was able to fight off that middle-age spread by watching my diet. The hard work paid off. Some eighteen years after my first pregnancy, I finally made my way back to my original pre-pregnant size. That summer I went out shopping for a bikini (something I hadn't worn since high school) and was delighted when the young salesgirl commented on my "six-pack." I felt great, looked great, and easily ignored the varicose veins, stretch marks, and cellulite on my butt and thighs. I'd reached my own goal of physical fitness and was proud of my accomplishment.

My boobs, though, were another story. They'd been a source of awkwardness my entire life. First they were too big (a DD in high school), then gargantuan during my pregnancies. By the time I'd finished nursing my third child, they'd lost all volume and lay flat against my chest. No one else would have known about their sad appearance, since they were easily camouflaged by foam bras capable of propping up anything one might choose to put on her chest. My husband still found me exciting and attractive and had accepted my body's many physical transformations during our twenty-two-year marriage. But having achieved my peak physical condition—when I finally liked how my butt, thighs, arms, and stomach looked in a swimsuit—I realized there was nothing I could do to physically improve my breasts. There was no exercise, no diet, no expensive cream that would make my breasts "fit," or at least complement my more well-toned self.

I'd never considered plastic surgery as an option. I figured it was only for women who wanted their breasts enlarged, or reduced. I wasn't too big (I wore a 36C bra, which I later discovered was the wrong size) and didn't care to be bigger. Then, one day I was shopping for a dress in my friend's clothing store. I thought I'd found the perfect flattering frock—except when it came to an ill fit in the bust. My girlfriend called in the alterations person to try and engineer some bralike support. Frustrated with the extra time and effort being made, I started complaining out loud about my boobs. My good friend rolled her eyes at me and asked, "If you're so unhappy, why not get a breast lift?"

After much research, that's just what I did. I interviewed three different physicians, all of whom had their own opinion about what I should or shouldn't choose to do with my breasts. Two of them thought I'd be unhappy with a simple lift and suggested I add small implants to regain my lost volume. I didn't take their advice for a number of reasons—among them the additional cost and complications associated with implants and my own family history of breast cancer.

My decision was not made to please my partner, either. He was opposed to the surgery, telling me repeatedly that it wasn't something he thought I needed. He wasn't thrilled about the idea of my having

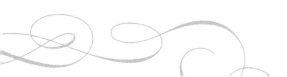

"unnecessary" surgery. He did agree to meet with my doctor and discuss the possible risks and complications. In the end, though, he knew it was a decision only I could make for myself.

Did I get perfect breasts? Yes and no. For the first time in my life, they fit with my body and are proportionate to my size. My areolae were made smaller, though I'm not thrilled with their new, cookie-cutter edges. My breasts have scars, and they're certainly not like the perky ones plastered all over Victoria's Secret ads (although I can fake that look with the right equipment). My 34C bras do fit better, since I'm no longer folding breast tissue into their cups. I can go bra-less if I want to, although my surgeon warned that too much of that would hasten inevitable breast sag. My girls are now more hassle-free. I no longer adjust my clothing choices to suit their shape and size. My breasts are much less important to me now than before my surgery. I have gained power over them, instead of feeling overpowered by them.

My surgery prompted me to look back at how my breasts had changed throughout my life. I began to write about their changes and talk with other women about breasts. I listened to their breast stories. I discovered that the true power of the breast rests in each of our unique bosoms.

BOTTOM BOOB LINE

We all have our own stories and experiences with our breasts. In these pages, you'll hear from experts and boob owners alike. You'll get advice from bra fitters, doctors, personal trainers, psychologists, and others. You'll learn how to meet your breast needs and how to overcome breast challenges. Women from all backgrounds share their "mammoirs" about the ups and downs of living with breasts. These mammoirs are the collective, universal story of our lives as women.

Breasts not only nurture our young, they can nurture us. They can be a source of enjoyment. We can look at ourselves in the mirror and think, *I am beautiful,* or feel completely the opposite. We can help our girls look better–or worse. We can decide to play them up as a physical asset or tone them down. We can use their power any way we choose. We can train our daughters to love their bodies and feel proud of their unique features. We can teach our sons that breasts are more than sex objects. Most of all, to truly know our breasts is to know ourselves. They are a living history on our chests. Our breasts need respect, care, love, and celebration. Let's give them what they deserve.

CHAPTER ONE

Bosom Buddies: Better Get to Know Your Girls

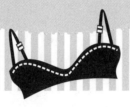

*The one thing I wish someone would have told me about my breasts
is that they would go from being an embarrassment to being a
point of pride to being an embarrassment again.*
—36C, AGE 56

*I'm in love with them. They fit in my hands and are decently symmetrical.
I love how soft and squishy they feel.
I wish I did have someone in my life to "share" them with.*
—32B, AGE 25

What qualities do you treasure in a close friend? A nurturing, supportive person who accepts both your virtues and flaws? Whatever your individual interests, you know each other well: likes, dislikes, even quirky yet endearing habits. You may not have known each other long, but you bonded instantly. And you can count on this friend in good or bad times. He or she will always be there for you, despite life's crazy ups and downs. This is the type of relationship you should have with your breasts. The body parts nearest to your heart should be thoroughly understood and accepted rather than discounted or ignored. Don't take them for granted, either, since your understanding of them will change over time. Care for them as you would your best buddy, and you'll have an enduring and healthy relationship for years to come.

Our breasts are wondrous orbs that define us as women, yet don't completely define who we are. They have been idealized, sexualized, and immortalized in art. They attract the opposite sex with little aid. Their preferred shape and size changes with fashion. Complex in nature, they are both sensual and functional. Some women carry them proudly; others feel more ashamed. Some of us don't think twice about our breasts, while other women obsess over self-perceived flaws. We all have breasts, and yet we relate to them in our own special way.

One thing's for sure: There's more to breasts than meets the eye. Even if we skipped basic breast anatomy, we'd fill more than one book on how they've been portrayed in history, art, politics, and language (see the Boobliography in the appendix). Then there's our personal view of our breasts—whether good, bad, or ambivalent. Or the constant but sometimes conflicting reports we read about breast-feeding, breast cancer, or general breast health. And we can't *un*cover all sides of our subject without taking a peek at society's present airbrushed vision of ideal breasts. Who knew there was so much to know about boobs?

To achieve complete breast understanding, you need to first measure your present bust knowledge. There's a lot that most of us don't know. Consider where you learned about average breast size, appearance, or biology. Was it from a friend, parent, doctor, teacher, or lover? Maybe everything you know today was discovered by watching TV, flipping through magazines, cruising the Internet, or sitting through some old movie in grade school. Whatever you learned may have at times seemed contradictory. For instance, some people think bras help prevent breasts from sagging; others think they may cause cancer. And that's just on the topic of what we wear! You may fully appreciate that the primary biological purpose of our breasts is to feed children, yet still feel uncomfortable when you see a mother nursing in public. You may understand boobs' appeal in selling everything from porn to pasta, but feel offended when some stranger stares at your own rack. In fact, our boobs are more complicated than they look.

Breasts have been viewed throughout history in many different ways. Some cultures celebrated the breast as a symbol of fertility and abundance. This had nothing to do with size but everything to do with milk production. Breasts were worshipped for their power to feed or sustain life. Present society's preference for hiding certain parts of breasts (nipples), and highlighting others (cleavage), is far removed from ancient customs. Throughout most of history, women bared their breasts. It simply made sense in ancient cultures for continuously pregnant and lactating women to keep a baby's primary food source handy. Turning back the boob clock further, to the Minoans of 1700 BC, we find women wearing clothing that purposely exposed and exhibited their breasts (some even consider these garments the first bra). This wasn't done as some sexual turn-on, but as a symbol of supremacy. Representations of the revered goddesses of fertility often featured multiple breasts jutting from their upper torsos.

WHAT'S YOUR BOOB I.Q.?

Whether you've lived with your breasts for years—or you're just now budding—whatever your size, shape, or color, your boobs are yours and yours alone. So how well do you know them?

1. What's the ideal female body type portrayed in most modern media advertising?
   A small breasts, thin body **B** large breasts, thin body
   C large breasts, big booty

2. Breasts are mostly made up of which of the following?
   A mammary glands or milk ducts **B** muscle **C** fat

3. At what age do women achieve their full breast growth?
   A twenties **B** teens **C** after pregnancy

4. How many women buy bras without trying them on?
   A 15 percent **B** 38 percent **C** 51 percent

5. The average woman will wear how many different bra sizes in her lifetime?
   A three **B** six **C** eight

6. How many women suffer breast pain when jogging?
   A 22 percent **B** 45 percent **C** 56 percent

7. What do American women most want in a bra?
   A comfort **B** style **C** nipple coverage

8. What is a "chicken cutlet"?
   A boneless chicken breast
   B a modern day version of the "falsie" **C** a new sexual position you'd like to try if your partner were willing

9. How often are women's breasts found to be symmetrical?
   A rarely   **B** somewhat often   **C** very often

10. What percentage of cosmetic breast augmentation (implant) surgeries in the U.S. are performed on eighteen- to nineteen-year-old women?
    A 3 percent   **B** 10 percent   **C** 25 percent

11. When pregnant, how many cup sizes will the average woman's breasts increase?
    A one   **B** two   **C** none

12. In what year did only five states in the U.S. have legislation protecting the rights of mothers to breastfeed in public?
    A 1974   **B** 1984   **C** 1994

13. At what age should a woman begin breast self-exams?
    A twenty   **B** thirty   **C** at puberty

14. What percentage of all breast cancers do mammograms detect?   **A** 80 percent   **B** 90 percent   **C** 100 percent

15. In what year were insurance companies required by law to pay for breast reconstruction after mastectomy?
    A 1972   **B** 1985   **C** 1999

16. How many days in a row should you wear the same bra?
    A one   **B** two   **C** five

17. Menopause causes women's breasts to do what?
    A increase in size   **B** decrease in size   **C** depends on the woman

18. What percentage of women who develop breast cancer have no family history of the disease?
    A 45 percent   **B** 60 percent   **C** 80 percent

FIND THE ANSWERS TO THESE QUESTIONS AND WHAT YOUR SCORE SAYS ABOUT YOUR BREAST KNOWLEDGE IN THE NAKED TRUTH, P. 235

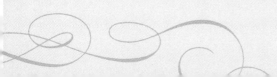

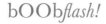

bOOb*flash!*

**WHAT DO BOOB ADMIRERS KNOW ABOUT
BREASTS THAT BOOB OWNERS DON'T?**

All breasts are unique and wonderfully different. Many of our lovers have viewed more than one pair on an intimate level. Ask yours if he or she has ever seen two exactly the same.

Greek statutes depicted torsos of small-breasted women. Other artists at other times (think Rubens) favored the more full-bosomed. As styles changed, so did the shape of breasts. They have been pushed up high by corsets, flattened low in tight bodices, pointed straight out in bullet brassieres, and pulled together tightly in wonder-how-they-do-that bras. It's easier to look at them from every perspective, really, but our own.

BOOBS 101

Breasts are like avocados: At twenty, they aren't quite ripe, at thirty they're perfect, and at forty they are overly ripe.

—36B, AGE 44

It's no wonder women struggle to find proper support for their breasts. There isn't a typical breast to which we can compare ourselves. "The wide range in size and shape of breasts makes it hard to say what's 'normal,'" writes Dr. Susan M. Love in her book *Dr. Susan Love's Breast Book.*[1] Whatever your breast size, however ideal or unusual they may appear to you, they are—in reality—the perfect breasts. It turns out that our girls are a lot like us: ever changing, adaptable, and totally unique.

It's unclear why human breasts evolved differently from other mammals', which develop only when lactating. In fact, human mammals are the only species to carry around fully formed breasts when *not* producing milk. Scientists have been debating this mystery for years. There is the upright, butt-cleavage theory espoused by Desmond Morris in *The Naked Ape*,[2] which states that the male's fixation on women's breasts can be linked to his former attraction for the female walking-on-all-fours backside. Then there's the hairless-human-body theory, which proposes that without any hair to cling to, pendulous breasts gave babies something to hang on to when nursing.[3] Still others speculate that extra fat stores helped women survive through multiple childbirths.[4] Finally, and my personal favorite, is the aqua-woman hypothesis. This one originates from the notion that hairless human beings were once underwater creatures, and breasts served as an infant's built-in life preserver.[5] The debate about whether women's breasts evolved as signals to lovers, food for babies, or for our own well-being may never be resolved.

Beautiful and mesmerizing, breasts are an amazing feat of engineering. They have no muscles, yet stand at attention. They also contain an intricate ductal system designed to produce and deliver the ideal food for a newborn. The breast itself encompasses a large part of our upper-body territory. Each extends from underneath the clavicle (or collarbone) down to the ribs and from the middle of our chest to the backs of our armpits.[6] That's a lot of geography to cover during a monthly breast self-exam.

What exactly are breasts? Because they're named "mammary glands," (derived from "mama," a baby's usual first word for mother), we might assume that's their total composition. But they're made up mostly of fat, which explains their changing size when we gain or lose weight. Breasts form in utero, around the sixth week of life. They follow a path along what's called the "milk ridge," a line that forms from our armpits to our groin area. Other mammals keep this

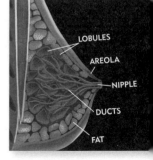

Véronique Estiol/Photo Researchers, Inc.

LOBULES
AREOLA
NIPPLE
DUCTS
FAT

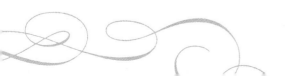

milk ridge, which is why they have more than two nipples. By the ninth week of gestation, this area in humans is contained within the chest region. Often, a newborn—of either sex—will leak "witch's milk" from its nipples. This scary-sounding substance is merely the breasts' response to a mom's hormones and disappears shortly after birth.

In women, it isn't until puberty that hormones again trigger breast growth. Within our buds grows an array of individual milk-producing glands, all converging at the nipple. Surrounding this system are the connective tissue and ligaments that hold everything in place. Breasts contain no muscle, except the underlying pectoral muscles (discussed in Chapter 9: Your Breast Potential). It is the very fine Cooper's ligaments that hold everything else up, most of the time. Some experts theorize that women's heavy reliance on bras may lead to the atrophy of these ligaments and hinder their natural ability to keep our breasts aloft.

Breast skin elasticity is also genetically determined. (If our peaches plummet, we can blame our DNA.) Some breasts are lumpy; some breasts aren't. Most women have nipple hair. Some have nipples that face frontward, although most face to the side. The areola contains a miniature smooth muscle that forces our nipples to stand at attention when stimulated sexually or due to nursing or a cold shot of air. Ever notice little bumps on your areola? Those are the sebaceous, or oil, glands. They contain natural lubricants to protect our nipples when nursing. Areolae come in a variety of shapes, sizes, and colors. They can be light or dark and can change color and shape during sexual arousal and pregnancy.

Nipples also come in an assortment of shapes and sizes. Some are flat, inverted, or stick out. They change size and color before and after pregnancy, and then again in menopause. Some women (and men) have "extra" nipples left over from our ancestral milk ridge. These can look like moles or other small bumps and may even lactate when a woman is nursing. Breastmilk doesn't spurt out in one big stream, like it does through a baby bottle. It travels through several milk duct openings. Some women may be concerned that their breasts should be bigger in order to nurse, but there's no evidence it makes any difference. Some nipple shapes may make nursing more difficult, but there are ways to overcome those problems successfully (see Chapter 7: Fully Employed Boobs).

"No other organ, apart from the uterus, changes so dramatically in size, shape, and function as the breast does during puberty, pregnancy, and lactation," writes Natalie Angier.[7] Hormone swings drive this steady state of flux. That's why our breasts feel heavier right before our periods, increase in size during pregnancy, and then sometimes shrink in volume after menopause. If men were given the same hormones women naturally produce during pregnancy, they too could breastfeed. (Maybe then breastfeeding in public might be a nonissue.) Whether large or small, breast size has nothing to do with milk production. We all have the same relative amount of milk-producing tissue; it's the added fat that creates proportional discrepancies.

No two breasts are exactly alike, even on the same woman. One may be bigger or higher or lower, with nipples pointing in different directions. Think yours aren't distinctive? Examine your ears, feet, or even eyes. Small differences can be found in any two similar physical features we possess. Check out your naked body in the mirror and you'll discover two comparable, yet different, boobs. The only twin girls we'll ever see are those perfected by a plastic surgeon, and even those will have some noticeable scars.

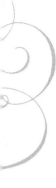

POWER TOOLS

My friends and I have always compared our breasts with each other's.
I call mine "little guys" . . . while another girlfriend—who is an F—tells
me I can have ALL of hers. All my small-chested friends want big
boobs, and vice versa. It's funny how that always turns out.

−34B, AGE 23

Breasts are powerful. They also exert influence over you, the boob holder. More than just treating you to some cyclical soreness, your breasts can color your view on life. Studies show that, for women, a negative body image is linked to low self-esteem. Our view of our bodies is no trivial matter. It can lead to depression, poor job performance, and/or anxiety, just to name a few responses to these feelings. Low self-esteem is a factor in eating disorders, such as bulimia and anorexia nervosa.[8] Researchers have found that negative body image is typically associated with identifying one or more body parts as too big. But in studies involving women's dissatisfaction with their own breasts, perceptions of oneself as too big *or* too small correlated with lower self-esteem.[9] Either extreme makes us unhappy. Just goes to show that beauty does rest in the eye of the boob-holder.

No one's perfect. That's a fact. So let's stop expecting the same thing from our breasts. They're mostly masses of fat and tissue. Period. No different from that stuff on our thighs, but more sexually charged. It doesn't help to compare ourselves to unrealistic (yeah, yeah, we know) female media images. But we do. Studies show that women feel angrier and more depressed after looking at photos of digitally perfected female fashion models.[10] And they don't even have to be selling us clothes (or handbags or shoes). We like our bodies less no matter what's being sold in the ad.[11]

No one is immune to this "beauty and the breast" syndrome. Hollywood stars even have their girls enhanced without a visit to their plastic surgeon. Keira Knightley's breasts suddenly grew bigger in the *King Arthur* movie poster, all the way up to a C cup (she objected to an earlier version making them look like EEs). In a 2006 *Elle* interview, Knightley recounted how, on another shoot, an unnamed American magazine claimed its market research found that women prefer to see nothing smaller than a C cup on other women. Knightley thought it was crazy, but the periodical inflated her boobs for that cover as well.[12] In the United States, we've developed a one-size-fits-all breast mentality. And if the picture doesn't meet this breast expectation, we'll have it Photoshopped, thank you.

These perfected media images may contribute to our longing for something we don't have. Straight hair if ours is curly. Long legs if ours are short. Blue eyes if ours are green. And the developing breast is an easy first target for our adolescent obsessions. If they're thought too small, we stuff our bras with Kleenex. If they seem too big, we hide behind oversize sweatshirts and heavy sweaters, no matter the outside temperature. There's rarely a Goldilocks stage when we find them "just right" (and if they are, it's usually observed in hindsight). You may be convinced that you were shorted (or overly favored) in your breast inheritance. Looking in the bathroom mirror, you may judge yourself either too round, too flat, too big, too small, too lumpy, too firm, too saggy, or too _____ (fill in you own personal favorite). This limited view of your own girls doesn't tell the whole story, though. When you do this, you're only comparing yourself to one static view of your boobs. You may just be having a bad breast day. And when you get up tomorrow morning, they'll look different than they did yesterday, or ten months from now, and certainly ten years into the future.

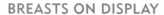

BREASTS ON DISPLAY

If we see only airbrushed breasts in comparison to a steady diet of movie and magazine breasts, our own real breasts don't fare so well. We simply don't see stretch marks, nipple hair, mastectomies, or lopsided, saggy breasts.

—MEEMA SPADOLA, *BREASTS: OUR MOST PUBLIC PRIVATE PARTS*[13]

What Spadola says here is true. All we see in movies, magazines, and on the boob tube are perky, petite, or too-big breasts. And what's with all the cleavage? Some scientists believe the cleavage attraction stems from our long lost walking-on-all-fours ancestors, who needed no pendulous protrusions to elicit male desire. In his 1967 book, *The Naked Ape,* Desmond Morris postulates that a woman's derriere was once viewed as a symbol of her fertility, making her more sexually desirable. Wide, fleshy hips signaled to the male of the species that the female was built for breeding. When we began to walk upright, that strong visual aid disappeared and our current forward-facing appendages evolved.[14] Voila, cleavage obsession was born. The sexual green light of our times is two breasts tightly pressed together. And since sex sells, these shelves of breasts are called upon to continuously promote products throughout the land.

The average person sees three to five hundred ads per day,[15] and it's been estimated that if you live to the ripe young age of sixty, you'll see forty to fifty million ads in your lifetime. Women repeatedly shown images of the currently in vogue, überthin female body standard, versus noncommercial everyday images, do experience more stress, anger, anxiety, and depression.[16] Naturally, a woman who sees hundreds and thousands of the popular and in-demand C cup breasts can't help but compare them to her own. But the boob truth is that these breasts on display are not representative of real, average women.

With so many naturally occurring variations it would be difficult, if not impossible, to determine an "average" breast size. Whether that's the one splashed across the covers of most lifestyle—and men's—magazines is debatable. Unfortunately, there are no reliable scientific studies measuring women's breast sizes. The only way to gauge averages may be to track sales of specific bra sizes. Swimsuit and lingerie models seem to stay in the 32B to 34C range (the "C" cup representing the voluptuous standard). Is that what we should assume is "normal"?

Not according to bra fitters and buyers in major department stores. Inflation has hit the bra business. Women's breasts have gotten bigger and bustier in the last ten to fifteen years. Industry reports on larger-bra sales prove this trend is here to stay. The full-figure classification (D to DDD range and above) started growing in the early 1990s and is still booming.[17] Despite what you might think, this trend isn't due to an increase in elective breast surgeries (see Chapter 11: Cut and Paste).

Girls are simply developing breasts earlier, and getting larger. Training bras once sold to thirteen- and fourteen-year-old girls are now being bought by eight- and nine-year-olds. And the United States is not alone in this busting-out-all-over phenomenon. A European marketing survey shows that almost 30 percent of Dutch women in the thirty to thirty-nine age group wear a D cup size or larger.[18] The cause is not clear. Some experts think birth control pills and animal hormones in food are to blame. Others believe it may be due to environmental factors or increased breast augmentations. Since breasts are made up mostly of fat, the real culprit may be the rise of obesity in the general population. A recent report stated that bra producers in China have been forced to offer bigger cup sizes because women there "are eating more nutritiously."[19] Whatever the reason, many women are baffled by this trend. They prefer to believe bra sizes are shrinking (more on that in Chapter 2: Bras) rather than accept the fact that breasts are expanding.

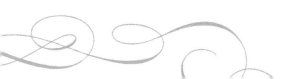

BOOB LINGO

Has any other body part possessed so many monikers? Nicknames for breasts vary as much as the appendages themselves. These affectionate examples speak to the joys of breast discourse: bazooms, beauts, big brown eyes, bombshells, boobies, boobs, bosom, bra buddies, breasticles, bubbies, bust, cha-chas, cushions, fun bags, gazongas, girls, happy bags, headlights, headrests, highbeams, hooters, joy toys, knockers, mounds, num-nums, pillows, sweater kittens, ta-tas, tits, the twins, and ya-yas.

According to etymologists, the word "boob" originated as slang for breasts in 1929. But the word "booby" (from the fifteenth century) is the name assigned to a not-so-smart species of bird. One who acted like a "dumb bird" was often called a "boob." No one knows why this fowl word became affixed to a woman's bosom. Perhaps the word "boob" took on the moniker of a foolish or silly (usually) male because that's how some react to the sight of breasts. (For more examples of how each generation has made its own contributions to this boob vernacular, see the sidebar Boob Jargon.)

Breast idioms continue to convey mixed messages. Some celebrate the breast, while others are considered obscene. In July 1972,

BOOB JARGON: THEN AND NOW

Booby n. pl. boobies [modif. of sp. Bobo, fr. L balbus stammering, prob. of imit. origin] (1602) 1: an awkward foolish person: dope 2: any of several tropical seabirds (genus Sula) of the gannet family[20]

Booby hatch n. (1840) 1: a raised framework with a sliding cover over a small hatch on a ship 2: a psychiatric hospital[21]

Booby trap n. (1850) 1: a strap for the unwary or unsuspecting: pitfall 2: a concealed explosive device contrived to go off when some harmless-looking object is touched [22]

Booby prize n. (1889) 1: an award for the poorest performance in a game or competition 2: an acknowledgment of notable inferiority[23]

Boob n. (1909) 1: an ignorant or foolish person [syn.: dumbbell, dummy, dope, booby, pinhead] 2: either of two soft, fleshy milk-secreting glandular organs on the chest of a woman v: commit a faux pas or a fault or make a serious mistake; "I blundered during the job interview" [syn.: sin, blunder, goof][24]

Booboisie n. [blend of boob and bourgeoisie] (1922): the general public regarded as consisting of boobs[25]

Boob tube n. (1966): television[26]

Boobvious n. (2006): to blatantly stare at a woman's breasts[27]

Booblivious n. (2006): to be so distracted by the presence of breasts that you do not respond even when called by name[28]

Boobsketball n. (2006): cleavage catch, a game in which you try to throw various small objects down a woman's cleavage[29]

comedian George Carlin was arrested for saying the word "tits" (among other words deemed indecent) in a monologue satirizing the seven "dirty words" that could not be said on television. In 1978, the Supreme Court found Carlin's speech was protected under the First Amendment, long after the album on which he recorded the

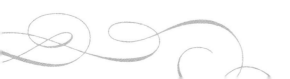

monologue went gold.[30] Once banned from speech (and definitely from view, as Janet Jackson's 2004 Super Bowl wardrobe malfunction proved), "tit" has generated a swelling list of positive illiterations: titalize, titulous, titastic, titilicious, titerrifc, and titacular.[31]

PUT YOUR BEST BREAST FORWARD

One woman may not have the power to change her culture's narrow view of breasts, but she can change her own. Embrace your boobs from a new direction! Instead of always looking down, try to view them from as many angles as your multidimensional wonders deserve. Check out these ways to better understand and know all breasts, or make up your own.

ACCEPT EVER-CHANGING STYLES

This decade's "in" boob look is next decade's "out" fashion style. Bra styles change continually (see Chapter 2: Bras), while boob biology remains constant. Empire waists, plunge V-necks, sweater sets, tank tops, and feminine, frilly blouses all go in and out of favor with designers. Find one look that fits your girls best, and feel good about how you look. And, please, spend some time reading Chapter 2, on how to buy and care for the right-size breast wardrobe.

SURVEY YOUR BREAST FRIENDS

Next time you get together with a group of gals, whether on vacation or an all-women work retreat, *notice* their breasts. You don't need to stare, but just acknowledge variations. Look around the room and see if you can't make a mental note of how many differences there are in size, shape, or color. You can play this game at parties, while shopping for groceries, or even walking around the mall or jogging down the street. Reminding yourself of how real women with real bodies look helps balance the visual scale of breast images. What is "normal" suddenly takes on new shape.

OPEN YOUR EYES TO PLAIN, BUT NOT SIMPLE, BOOBS

Visit a gym or all-women's spa and you'll (a) release your own inhibitions by revealing your breast bod, and (b) realize that each woman is a marvelous and individual creation. Better yet, get yourself to a topless swimming spot and take in the diversity on display. You don't have to visit the French Riviera either. Topless beaches in Canada and the United States, and some hotels in Las Vegas, now offer European sunbathing at their resorts.

If you're uncomfortable baring your own, there are plenty of fine photography books and nonporn Internet sites that celebrate our girls' differences. Visit 007 Breasts' photo gallery[32] or other websites and books listed in the Boobliography. These regular-gal pics remind you that you'll never find a pair quite like your own.

DECLARE YOUR LOVE AND ADMIRATION

Tell your girls you love 'em—and not just when you're naked or on a day when you're admiring how they look. Thank them for their unlimited potential. Though you may not be a woman who's going to watch them transform through pregnancy or use them to nurse, you can still give them kudos for hanging in there. And don't ignore your best friend's rack either! Spread some praise when she radiates both inner and outer beauty in a cute outfit.

MAKE A PLAY DATE WITH YOUR GIRLS

Do more than the ordinary with your extraordinary set. Create a "tit print" in the snow on a winter's day or in the warm sand of a sunny beach. Take your girls out for a spin in a burlesque-themed tassel-twirling class. Or just come home after work, strip off the old bra, and let them hang out with you on the couch while watching a movie.

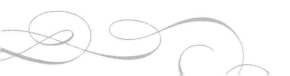

CHAPTER TWO

Bras:
Getting the
Breast Fit

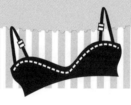

I think the whole science of bra engineering is like so many things: If men had to wear 'em, these problems would have received more attention long ago.
—36C, AGE 56

It is hard to find a bra for very small breasts! I know many people complain that they have trouble wearing bras if they are too big—and my problem is just the opposite. I need the right amount of padding so that it doesn't look too fake or so I don't look flat as a wall.
—32A, AGE 28

A bra can be a girl's best friend, or her worst enemy. This often has little to do with whether one undergarment fits better than another. We often choose style over support. But that's not so unusual. Many women buy a gorgeous pair of shoes knowing that it has a cruel heel or scrapes against their big toe. But it doesn't matter, because this must-have footwear has another, more important purpose: It accentuates the shape of our legs, or matches perfectly with some ensemble we own. We accept the fact that we don't always buy shoes for comfort. Even when we choose something reserved for sporting activities, we still want them to *look* good. We don't often get that magic combination of appeal and comfort in the same bra package. And when we do, it seems we pay a mighty high price for a wee bit of material that very few people ever see. And some of the most fashionable bras look worse once we've covered them up with our clothing. It's not as though we get a guaranteed fit when we do spend more on our intimate apparel. Unlike in other areas of the clothing industry, it's not easy to just go out and buy a custom-made bra or have the ones we own altered to meet our specific physiques. We are normally left to buy "off the rack" for our racks.

HANG 'EM HIGH

Lift and shape—that's all we really want in a bra. Get those bosoms where fashion says they ought to be, or perhaps where they once were. Pull them out from under your armpits and move 'em front and center. Get the loose skin pushed up a little higher so you'll look great in your clothes. But what about comfort? Knowing that women seek comfort *and* style in their foundations, the highly competitive bra industry attempts to meet this simple goal every year. And yet, truly comfortable and stylish bras seem to elude women everywhere. After all, what happens when you open your lingerie or underwear drawer in the morning? Do you grab the first bra you see with the confident, cool knowledge that it's a perfect fit, that it will make you look and feel your very best?

No. In all likelihood, you wade through an array of multisize bras that you bought for any number of reasons. You find the "special occasion" bra—the one purchased for a particular outfit that you haven't worn since. You may reluctantly push aside your comfy sports bras (secret favorites, yes, but unsuitable for anything other than athletics or lounging around on the weekends). Finally, you reach for whatever bra you guess makes you look best. It's probably a year or two old. Maybe you look at the tag and think to yourself, *Hey, wait a minute. My girls are a C?* Maybe every single bra you own appears defective: too much or too little padding, painfully tight cups or underwire, pinching or slipping straps. You know your body too well to have bought something that doesn't fit, don't you? It might be easier to blame any discomfort on our breasts instead of the bra. But it's generally not their fault.

"Did you know that 85 percent of all women wear the wrong-size bra?" asked bra fitting expert Susan Nethero in her appearance on *The Oprah Winfrey Show*.[1] Why is this the case? First, your boobs are as different from the next woman's as your DNA. Even if you are the exact same bust size as the woman standing next to you, it's unlikely you wear the exact same bra. Nor should you. Victoria Roberts, owner of Zovo Lingerie says: "I could have ten 32D women in one room and each might fit in a different bra."[2] Breast fullness, softness, and tautness of skin (and where it falls) make bra fitting a true art form. No wonder we struggle to find the right size!

We too often forget that our breasts are in a constant state of flux. Experience a weight gain (or loss) of ten pounds and you'll be a different cup size. Start (or quit) an exercise routine and watch your breasts react. Age a few years and gravity does another number on you. Some women's boobs make more dramatic changes than others. Don't worry. You're not alone. Most women don't realize that their girls are constantly shifting: Get your period, go on or off the pill, have babies, nurse, have another baby, go through menopause, et cetera, et cetera—all of it impacts your breast size.

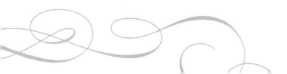

And our tastes change, too. In our twenties we want the latest fashion, the cutest bra. As we get older, our bra preferences also shift. Many of us choose practical comfort over the latest bra trends. And since most of us gain a bit of weight and see the redistribution of our boob flesh as we age, it comes as no surprise that boomers are driving the demand for larger-size bras.[3] One interesting study showed that plenty of women stop wearing bras altogether as they get older. It found that half of women age fifty and up preferred being braless, and 20 percent no longer wear bras at all![4] Maybe the more years we spend wearing these devices the more fed up we are with the entire process. Even those of us who haven't abandoned the quest for support are probably neglecting to update our selection of bras. We avoid professional fittings and stuff our bosoms into uncomfortable, yet familiar, brassieres.

THE RISE OF AN UPLIFTING INDUSTRY

I hate having to wear them, I hate that they never fit, and
I hate how you have to go through this ridiculous routine to be fitted
for a bra. Why does someone have to come into this tiny dressing room,
where I'm invariably sweaty, make me lift my arms, put a sticky tape
measure around me, and then pronounce to the world my size?
—38C, AGE 46

The earliest ancestor of today's contemporary bra first appeared in the mid-1800s. Promoted as a healthier alternative to the corset (not to mention less constricting), these "breast supporters" were designed and patented by both men and women.[5]

The term "brassiere" was first used in 1904 by the Charles R. DeBevoise Company. Despite its health-conscious origins, health was soon compromised as fashion began to drive brassiere styles. The popularity of the cinched-in corseted look led to ever more slimming lines in bra design as well.[6]

When the flapper era arrived in the 1920s, women bound their breasts to look flat in straight, columned dresses. Ironically, during those years, manufacturers began to design brassieres for a range of differently endowed customers. The first "uplift" models appeared in 1923; fabric shaped into "cups" followed in 1927. One "bust confiner," patented specifically for larger women, appeared to be one solid piece of fabric gathered in the center of the chest with no defined and separate band. Bras were primarily sold by catalog, and companies used the size designations Small, Medium, Large, and Stout (some makers held to these terms until the 1940s). Innovations continued (including the first post-mastectomy bra in 1918), but alphabet cup sizing and adjustable straps were not introduced until the mid-1930s.[7]

These early bra beginnings were driven in part by an ever-growing market for the brassiere, prompting market innovations and the introduction of new materials, such as elastics, into the industry. Women who once made their own bras at home began to rely on mail-order catalogs to furnish them with affordable undergarments. And while some women might want to blame the invention of the underwire bra on some non–boob owner (or a real "boob" of a guy), it was actually patented by Madelaine Gabeau in 1911.[8] After World War II, when wire became more affordable, underwire bras became the standard in the industry. Stretchable fabrics also permitted the creation of multisize bands. The postwar baby boom ushered in the development of maternity and nursing bra lines. Necessity, not always fashion, was another driving force behind bra inventions.

Although some of these advances did result in increased comfort and support, fashion prompted most of the brassiere's biggest changes. The 1930s saw hemlines rise, waists reappear, and a return to the look of full breasts. (Imagine the shock to small-busted women when the flattened bosom look of the 1920s went out of style in one short decade.) College girls aspired to wear a "sweater girl" and skirt uniform. By the 1940s, Hollywood brought bosomy, curvaceous women onto the

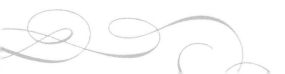

BRASSIERE INVENTORS OR IMPOSTERS?

Who invented the first noncorset device that most closely resembles our modern-day bra? Was it Otto Titzling, reputed to have lost a court battle over his original design to Phillip de Brassiere—which is why today's garment is called a brassiere, not a titzling? This charming story has its roots in the 1971 satire *Bust-Up: The Uplifting Tale of Otto Titzling and the Development of the Bra*, by Wallace Reyburn, and was further popularized in a 1985 song by Bette Midler.[9] Fortunately, or maybe unfortunately, there's no truth to this humorous story. The first use of the word "brassiere" (derived from the French/Norman word for "woman's bodice") is most often attributed to the Charles R. DeBevoise Company in 1904.[10] But patents for all kinds of "breast confiners" or "supporters" appeared in the late 1880s. Marie Tucek's push-up design of 1893, although never widely manufactured, closely resembles today's demibra.[11] In Paris, Herminie Cadolle, already in the corset-making business, unveiled her *le bien-être* ("the well-being") invention in 1889. In 1914, Mary Phelps Jacob claimed to be the inventor of the bra when she patented her "brassiere" creation.[12] No matter who came first, this new contraption found fast and widespread acceptance. By 1918, there were fifty-two brands of bras on the market.[13]

screen. From Mae West to Marilyn Monroe, boobs were definitely back in vogue. The 1940s also saw more women entering the workforce to support the war effort. Manufacturers met the challenge to support breasts despite war-related rubber shortages that reduced the quantity of elastic that was available. It would be logical to imagine that strapless, padded, push-up, and underwire bras would be put on the back burner in favor of more-practical choices, but that was not the case: Manufacturers instead increased their output of bras by 50 percent. By the 1950s, Frederick's of Hollywood had opened its first store, catering to the new sexy pinup-girl look.

By the 1960s, Twiggy was in; Jane Russell was out. In the '60s women threw out their bras, and in the '70s they shunned support altogether. How did bra manufacturers respond to this chaos? They presented a softer, more natural cup silhouette. Then clothing styles changed again. The '80s were all about BIG: shoulder pads, hair, and, yes, boobs. This decade also spawned the first wave of silicone implants (see Chapter 11: Cut and Paste).

The mid-1990s gave the bra industry its biggest boom. The Wonderbra was introduced, and with it cleavage was reborn. Even though Wonderbra's current design hit the market in 1964, it wasn't until the mid-1990s that this style became a media and marketing darling—thanks to the help of fashion magazines.[14] Soon competing manufacturers raced to produce their own versions, such as the Victoria's Secret Miracle Bra. Sex sells, and ads for these bras often seemed directed more to men than women, with cleavage being touted as the latest fashion accessory.

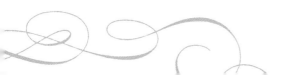

BEST-DRESSED BREASTS

I hate them! I don't care how much they cost, what brand they are—they are uncomfortable. Especially sports bras. The lacy ones look sexy but they are itchy, and you can't wear them under anything without showing. The straps always fall off my shoulders, so I have to wear racer backs, but those are hard to wear under tanks and sleeveless shirts. Plain ones for T-shirts feel ugly and boring.
—34B, AGE 37

So where are we today? Nowadays it's all about choice, ladies. You can buy your bras almost anywhere—from catalogs, department stores, the web, fashion designers, and lingerie boutiques. You can find bras in every style and shape and for nearly every occasion: push-ups, minimizers, strapless, backless, cross-in-the-back, long-line, underwire, soft cup, molded cup, even "pump 'em up" bras—not to mention every imaginable color, fabric, and style.

Yes, the bra industry is in great shape. In 2001, 396 million bras were sold in the United States alone, and sales of bras rose to $5.2 billion in 2005.[18] Half of all women purchase a bra every four to six months, and younger women purchase bras even more frequently. Women buy four to five bras each year, spending an average of $77 annually. Yet, seven out of ten women have never been professionally fitted.[19] In choosing a bra, many women treat their breasts with less respect than they do their feet. After all, it's common to have your feet measured, and most women have a clear sense of whether shoes fit when buying a new pair.

Bra manufacturers have also quickly adapted to the swelling-breast trend of the past ten to fifteen years. The fastest-growing market in intimate apparel is geared to bigger-breasted woman, with sales for larger sizes nearly twice what it is for smaller-breasted women.[20] Companies such as Vanity Fair and Olga, among other major brands, have all launched larger lingerie lines to meet this demand. New brands, such as Prima Donna and Panache, show their wares on plus-size lingerie models. And smaller manufacturers specializing in larger bra sizes have found their businesses booming as a result. At the 2006 Lingerie Americas trade show (one of the largest such trade fairs and now a triannual event), 72 of the 270 exhibitors offered their products in plus sizes. Bra marketers claim they are finally focusing on the needs of a population long ignored. But bra fitters believe the industry is merely responding to burgeoning bust lines due in part to rising rates of obesity.

Entrepreneur Jodi Gallaer, frustrated with trying to dress her own 32DDs, and equipped with an MBA from Harvard, started her bra business in 2005. Demand for her new larger line of lingerie more than doubled in its first year on the market, and she now carries sizes 28C to 40H.[21] This should be a great relief to busty women, whose choices have seemed limited through the years. Still, if you are an H cup or larger, you must go to a specialty store to find attractive bras

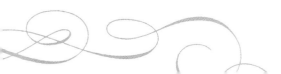

BACK IN STYLE: THE BUSTIER AND OTHER BODICES

Although the bra was first invented as a healthful alternative to the rib-crushing corset, the feminine silhouette of the bra's predecessors has not been lost on today's designers. Some historians believe that it's the corset's ability to hide our body's flaws—whether by creating the illusion of a smaller waist or pushing up our boobs—that's contributed to its ongoing popularity. And the bustier and corset have made a definite comeback—and not just in music videos and movies.

Today's boned bodices are more often than not purposely worn as "outerwear." The House of Cadolle (founded in the 1880s by Herminie Cadolle, often noted as the inventor of the bra) never abandoned the business of creating such one-of-a-kind custom designs for its exclusive clientele. Poupie Cadolle, the great-great-great-granddaughter of Herminie, offers her couture creations to those who can afford the very best. Mme. Cadolle believes that the 118-year tradition is still alive because "corsets are both glamorous and functional. They are beautiful and seductive, resculpting the natural curves of a woman, uplifting her bust, minimizing and flattering her body."[22]

Other manufacturers have caught on to this trend and now regularly feature bustiers or other bodices as part of their lines. (Check out the Boobliography for a listing of retailers.)

in your size. Macy's and Nordstrom carry some thirty different brands of bras between them, yet the largest is only a 46G. Victoria's Secret, with more than nine hundred retail stores across the country (plus its website), sells nothing bigger than a DD cup. (Check out the Boobliography in the appendix for additional solutions and resources for well-endowed women.)

Other accessories have cropped up to make our breasts look even better in our bras. Small-breasted women can buy bras designed to enhance their size or create cleavage. We can purchase "cookies" or silicone "cutlet" inserts to help even out the naturally uneven sizes of our breasts. These come in a variety of different shapes, sizes, and materials. There are tapes and stickers to cover too-rigid nipples, as well as fake plastic nipples that you can insert in your bra to produce a more revealing look. Band extenders provide a better fit for women with broad backs or with respiratory problems like asthma. You can even buy detachable fabric and crystal-encrusted bra straps to invigorate the look of your bra wardrobe.

The bra industry continues to stay on the cutting edge. Scientists are now working to develop the world's first "smart bra." This bra would sense when breasts are in motion and increase tightness and support in the band, cups, and straps in response.[23] (A *really* smart bra would also change colors to match our outfits!)

OUR CUPS RUNNETH OVER

I love the multitude of options with today's bras. I once tried on a bra that hoisted my boobs up so high, my chin was practically resting on them. . . . I did not purchase the bra. But strapless bras still suck, at least for my breasts. They are terribly uncomfortable and do a lousy job of keeping my boobs in place. They offer almost no support.

—36C/D, AGE 34

What do professional bra fitters say is the number one mistake women make when buying a bra? We buy them too large in the band and too small in the cup. We often think our breasts are held in place by the straps of our bra. In fact, the *band* is specifically engineered to carry the weight of our breasts. The straps are merely an adjustment tool. Why do we squeeze our breasts into smaller cups? That's harder to determine, but it may be because many of us don't believe in the true measure of our bosom. Rebecca Apsan, owner of La Petite Coquette in New York and author of *The Lingerie Handbook,* believes women are simply in a state of "bra cup denial." "They think their breasts will look huge, but as a matter of fact, it's the exact opposite. The right-size bra will empower them," says Apsan.[24]

We don't like to think of our breasts as "fat" (even though that's exactly what they are), so we squish our girls into places too small to be comfortable. Then we double our pain with too-taut straps that cut into our shoulders, leaving unsightly marks from trying to hold us up. Most bra fitters agree that going up a cup size and going down one band size is usually the first step to take when you feel uncomfortable in your bra.

BASIC BRA RULES

RULE #1: ACCEPT THAT YOUR BREASTS ARE SPECIAL

Accepting your size is the first step in finding a bra that not only fits, but fits well. Karen Bierwagen is a Le Mystère sales consultant who calls herself a "boobologist." She has seen plenty of breasts in her nearly two decades as a bra fitter. Bierwagen believes most women need to face reality when it comes to their true bra size. Women might think if they wear anything larger then the B and C cups featured in fashion magazines, there's something abnormal about their breasts. "The truth is that DD is closer to the average size of most women. So if you're a DDD, you're not far from the norm," says Bierwagen. Smaller women may be easier to fit, but they too can be dissatisfied with how their breasts appear.

Victoria Roberts, of Zovo Lingerie, believed she'd made a radical career change when she left her human relations position at Starbucks to go into the intimate apparel business. "It surprised me how much it's like my old job," she says. "I do more counseling in my fitting rooms then anything else. Women will apologize for their breasts no matter their size. But every woman is unique." Acceptance is the key.

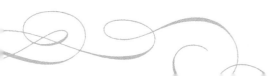

RULE #2: EXPECT DIFFERENCES IN BRA FITTERS

Some fitters take one or two measurements; others take three. Some department stores insist you wear a special "fitting" bra before you are measured. Others may not have dedicated fitting experts in every day. Some fitters have years of experience and are truly experts in their field. Selma Koch, who owned the world-renowned Town Shop in Manhattan and worked past her ninety-fifth birthday, only had to glance at a customer to determine her proper size. Rebecca Apsan, with thirty years experience, says she "never touched a tape measure," and instead relies on her own method of trial and error.[25]

RULE #3: ACCEPT THAT NOT ALL BRAS FIT ALIKE

Finding a bra that fits you well is not just about your distinct physical qualities. "There is no standard size in bra manufacturing," says Bierwagen of Le Mystère. (There's not even a professional lingerie association that could endorse or enforce such standards!) You may know your correct size, but you won't know how this corresponds to the sizing the various manufacturers use.

bOOb*flash!*

UNDERWIRE PAIN?

Any wire in your bra should encircle your entire breast. If not, it will end up pinching your breast tissue. A quick way to test potential comfort is to push your thumbs against the wires on the both sides of your bra. They should rest on the hard bone of your rib cage, not the soft flesh of your breasts.

This is why you should rely on the help of an experienced bra fitter. A pro will know. She'll be familiar with many manufacturers and their styles and be able to easily and quickly recommend the type of bra that fits your exceptionally beautiful and original breasts.

KNOW THY BREASTS, KNOW THY BRA

I spent what seemed like six hours in the dressing room, fighting hangers and hooks to buy "the perfect" new bra. While it seemed to fit in the store, it looked horrible at home. I'm either tightening the straps all the time or they slip off my shoulders constantly. I wish I could find my boobs a happy home.
—34B, AGE 34

First, take off your bra and look at yourself in the mirror. Without being critical, take a good look at how your breasts hang. Are they more vertical than horizontal? Does more of your breast flesh hang down than from side to side? As we age, our breast tissue moves farther back on our chests. Certain types of bras will fit you better depending on where most of your flesh is located. If your breasts are more side to side (horizontal), you will want a bra that can gather up the tissue and bring it to the middle. Try a balconnette, demicup, or deep-plunge bra. (This style also works well for women who wear

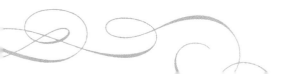

AA or AAA and find their girls swimming inside more-full-cup-style bras.) If your breast tissue hangs more vertically, you'll want a bra that pushes up your breasts from below.

If you're a B cup, you have the advantage of being able to choose from a variety of styles—or choose not to wear a bra at all (lucky girls). Women with C cups may not feel as comfortable going bra-less. Whether the majority of your breast tissue rests higher up on your chest or lower determines the bra that's best for your boobs. If you are a D cup or larger, consider wearing underwire bras for comfort and support. If you have had surgery on your breasts and are larger than a C cup, you may prefer a nonunderwire bra to reduce pressure on healing scar tissue. Many women with breast augmentations choose to wear shelf-bra camisoles for comfort. (For specific recommendations for sports and maternity bras, please see Chapter 6: Mammaries in Motion and Chapter 7: Fully Employed Boobs.)

THE MEASURE OF YOUR MAMMARIES

Most of them just seem to be so uncomfortable over long periods of time. I have a very hard time finding ones that fit me well, so I hate it when I have to buy them.

—38C, AGE 33

How do you determine your proper bra size? First, find a cloth tape measure (probably the hardest part of this task). Next, put on a bra (yes, I know, it sounds counterintuitive, but that's what experts recommend). Next, choose one of the following two methods:

1. Take two measurements—one under the bust circumference or at the rib cage (UTC), and the other across and over the boobs (OTB). The UTC is the number that determines your band size. The next step is to add five inches (but this number is not always consistent between bra manufacturers, fitters, and bra retailers) to the UTC number. Then subtract the UTC from the OTB to come up with another number that determines your bust size. For instance, a one-half- to one-inch difference is an A cup, a two-inch difference is a B cup, and so on.

2. Wrap the tape measure high around your back and bring it up across your breastbone above your breast tissue, giving you an over-OTB number. If the OOTB is an odd number, round it up to the next even number, then subtract that total from the UTC determined above. The number difference will correspond to the cup sizes referred to in paragraph 1 (one to one-half inch for an A cup, two inches for a B cup, et cetera).

The result is your cup size.

Your final number could also be flawed depending on whether you: (a) inhaled or exhaled while measuring; (b) measured yourself with your arms lifted or flat against the side of your body; or (c) had someone else take your statistics. This should make it clear why up to 85 percent of all women wear the wrong-size bra!

Los Angeles plastic surgeon Dr. Edward Pechter was so appalled by this system that he came up with what he believes is a much better

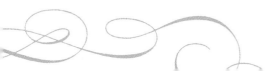

DR. PECHTER'S "SIZE ME UP" BRA SIZING CHART®

Breast width (in inches)

	5	5.5	6	6.5	7	7.5	8	8.5	9
27	32AA	32AA/A	32A	32A/B	32B	32B/C	32C	32C/D	32D
28	32AA	34AA	32A	34A	32B	34B	32C	34C	32D
29		34AA	34AA/A	34A	34A/B	34B	34B/C	34C	34C/A
30		34AA	36AA	34A	36A	34B	36B	34C	36C
31			36AA	36AA/A	36A	36A/B	36B	36B/C	36C
32			36AA	38AA	36A	38A	36B	38B	36C
33				38AA	38AA/A	38A	38A/B	38B	38B/C
34				38AA	40AA	38A	40A	38B	40B
35					40AA	40AA/A	40A	40A/B	40B
36					40AA	42AA	40A	42A	40B
37						42AA	42AA/A	42A	42A/B
38						42AA	44AA	42A	44A
39							44AA	44AA/A	44A
40							44AA	46AA	44A

method. "I found that the fault lies not with the women, but with the traditional method of bra measurement, which is highly inaccurate. Through my experience performing breast surgery, I have developed a bra measuring system to help women accurately find the correct bra size," says Dr. Pechter. His method consists of two calculations: the UBC (as above) and one that measures each breast separately, in their natural state of undress.

3. To find your UBC, wrap a tape measure snugly around your chest just under your breasts. To find your breast width (BW), measure across one breast on the side of the chest to where it ends next to the breastbone (passing over the nipple). Don't pull too hard or you'll compress the breast and get an incorrect reading. Small or firm

9.5	10	10.5	11	11.5	12	12.5	13	13.5	14
32D/DD	32DD	32DD/E	32E						
34D	32DD	34DD	32E	34E					
34D	34D/DD	34DD	34DD/E	34E					
34D	36D	34DD	36DD	34E	36E				
36C/D	36D	36D/DD	36DD	36DD/E	36E				
38C	36D	38D	36DD	38DD	36E	38E			
38C	38C/D	38D	38D/DD	38DD	38DD/E	38E			
38C	40C	38D	40D	38DD	40DD	38E	40E		
40B/C	40C	40C/D	40D	40D/DD	40DD	40DD/E	40E		
42B	40C	42C	40D	42D	40DD	42DD	40E	42E	
42B	42B/C	42C	42C/D	42D	42D/DD	42DD	42DD/E	42E	
42B	44B	42C	44C	42D	44D	42DD	44DD	42E	44E
44A/B	44B	44B/C	44C	44C/D	44D	44D/DD	44DD	44D/E	44E
46A	44B	46B	44C	46C	44D	46D	44DD	46DD	44E

breasts can be measured while standing, but large or droopy breasts are more accurately measured while lying down. Your breasts may each have a different measurement.

bOOb*flash!*

BRA CUPS ARE NOT CREATED EQUALLY

If you go *down* a band size in your bra, you should go *up* a size in the cup. For example, if you've been wearing a 34C that's too big in the band, you should move down a band size and up a cup, into a more comfortable 32D.

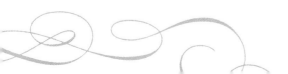

Next, find your UBC and BW numbers on Dr. Pechter's bra size calculator (see chart). The point where the two numbers intersect is your bra size. For example, if your UBC is 31 and your BW is 9, your bra size is 36C. A number like 36C/D means you fall between a C and a D cup in a size 36 bra, so you might fit one or the other, depending on the brand. If your UBC is between two numbers, for example 31.5, you can calculate your size for either 31 or 32 inches. Similarly, if your BW is between two numbers, for example 9.25, you can calculate your size for either 9 or 9.5 inches. Since all bra sizes differ, depending on style and manufacturer, Dr. Pechter's system isn't perfect, but he believes you can find your correct size 90 percent of the time.

IF THE BRA DON'T FIT, MUST YOU SUBMIT?

We live in the age of modern technology. It's time to get some true tech support for our breasts. Let's upgrade our software and toss those old floppies in the trash (or shred them if you like). Here's how:

GET FIT

Invest some time in your own comfort by being professionally fitted at your local department store or at a specialty lingerie boutique. Make it a double date for your girls by bringing along your best bosom buddy. You can celebrate your girls together! If you don't have a store

---

CHRISTEN YOUR CUPS

Since bra designers label our breasts by cup size, how about adding inspiring definitions to uplift our girls? Next time you shop for a bra, tell the bra fitters you are a "size 36 double-D divine." Try these or create your own!

A=Awesome	E=Excellent	I=Inspiring
B=Beautiful	F=Fabulous	J=Just Right
C=Charming	G=Gorgeous	K=Kind
D=Divine	H=Heavenly	L=Lovely

near you, enlist the help of a friend or lover. Use a cloth tape measure and have pen and paper handy. Choose from one of the methods described earlier to find your correct size.

GET BUSY

Once you've determined your size, set aside an hour and go to a store that carries a variety of makes and models. (You can always look for better deals of the same brands online once you know what you like.) Pick at least six bras in your size (hey, you've tried at least that many shoes in one sitting). Remember that more than half of these bras won't fit perfectly (each bra style is slightly different), so please don't blame your girls. Follow these simple rules:

1. **Hook up.** Fasten your bra on the loosest (first) hook. As the bra wears and the fabric loosens, you'll still be able to adjust by using the second or third set of hooks.

2. **Fill up.** Lean over and make sure you've got all your tissue in the cups. Your breasts should fill up the cup, not spill out the top or the sides. Note: When trying on underwire bras, make sure the wire is sitting on your rib cage (bone), rather than your breast tissue. If the cups look wrinkled, try a smaller band size, not a smaller cup size, first. Do the same when not filling up the more padded bra styles.

3. **Strap up.** Adjust the straps so they are lying flat against your shoulders but are not indenting your skin. Remember that everyone has two different-size breasts, so you may need to adjust straps at differing levels. Note: If, after this step, your bra rides up in back, try a smaller-size band or loosen the straps.

4. **Stand up.** Turn sideways and look at yourself in the mirror. The back band of the bra should be at the very same level as the front of your bra. The center front of the bra should lie flat against and not pull away from your breastbone. If you rest the palm of your hand on your stomach, your breasts should be situated halfway between your shoulder and your elbow.

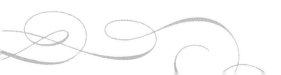

5. **Suit up.** Once you've found the right fit, re-dress for success! That's right, make sure you like the way the bra looks *underneath* your clothes. If you're not happy, you still have time to try on something that looks better.

6. **Match up.** Found a bra you love? Like the way it makes you look? Buy three or four pairs of underwear to complement its fabric or style. Don't go to all the trouble of making your girls looks good without remembering to properly accessorize!

BRA GATE: THE GREAT AMERICAN NIPPLE COVER-UP

According to lingerie fitters, American women prefer to keep flagrantly rigid nipples out of view. Whether they're stimulated by a chilly winter day or the overactive office AC, revealing this erect part of our anatomy just gives out too much information. We're happy with the ability to strap on a push-up bra for deep-cleavage special effects. But please, no nips.

In Europe this is a nonissue. Women there prefer to wear softer, lacier bras, ones that show more of the breasts' true form. Lingerie buyers estimate only 20 percent of all bra sales in Europe are of the molded cup variety, compared to 80 percent in the United States. And bra manufacturers know their markets. Walk through any U.S. Victoria's Secret or other favorite clothing retailer and you'll find racks and racks of these "McCups." They are the equivalent of Barbie boobs—hers being the first nip-less wonders.

So how do we make the most of this puritan modesty? Can we recycle these perky appliances and extend their half-life beyond local landfills? Let's think outside the bra! Turn them into wardrobe aids to hold socks and sachets. Or roll up matching panties inside for convenient safekeeping and storage. Outdoors, they can double as gardening kneepads. Wear them as earmuffs, kept secure by convenient hooks under our chin. Don't spend another dime on outdoor insulated faucet covers when a more convenient solution rests inside your home. These former bosom buddies can help fight flu epidemics if worn as personal mouth masks. (During a recent Asian SARS outbreak, bras were used in place of hard-to-find face masks.)[28]

No use is too fantastic. They can replace pesky packing peanuts or serve as the safest of Christmas ornament storage "chests." With the extra bun padding they give, you can enjoy an all-day bike ride. Sew them together to protect golf clubs, and add a button nose or eyes for a personal touch. We'll all be ready when shoulder pads come back in style. If nothing else, we can bare our imaginations.

BETTER BOOB WEAR PRINCIPLES

Both bra fitters and manufacturers applaud the well-fitting bra as a garment that can truly change a woman's life. But there's more to it then just dressing the girls right. You need to rotate and care for your lingerie properly. You'll not only get your money's worth, your purchases will last longer. After taking all the time and trouble to finally find what suits your girls best, why start all over again when you can practice some simple bra maintenance steps? The impetus for Jodi Gallaer starting her own bra business was her inability to outfit her own odd-size (by industry standards) girls in a fashionable way. Finding happiness in your lingerie isn't as shallow as its sounds. As Gallaer says, "No matter what you wear on the outside, you'll always feel like a rock star underneath." And no one deserves star treatment more than you and your girls!

Hopefully you'll be inspired to re-dress your girls by this point. Once you've become the proud owner of one well-fitting bra, put on your new purchase and take a good look at yourself in the mirror. Do you feel better? Do your girls look better? Go ahead and pat yourself on the back (or your chest). You'll have taken the very first step in learning to celebrate your girls. And remember to follow these simple steps in bra buying and maintenance for future purchases:

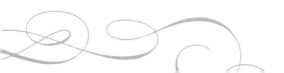

1. **Be honest.** Always ask yourself before you buy an outfit: Do I have the right underpinnings? That beautiful dress in the window may include the hidden cost of a new foundation. (Bra fitters comment that one of their more challenging customers is the bride-to-be. Typically, she picks out her dream gown: a gorgeous backless, strapless number. She strolls into the lingerie department and is startled to find her DDDs are an engineering challenge for her wedding dress.) Remember, you may have to invest more in a bra for the dress than in matching shoes or a handbag.

2. **Mark your calendar.** You've made a commitment to looking and feeling good, but you also have to keep up with the times. Don't assume because you've found a bra that fits you well that you can order any bra off the Internet in that *specific* size and live happily ever after. Schedule a fitting each year, just as you would a mammogram or PAP smear.

3. **Rotate for better wear.** Wearing a bra for two days and letting it rest for one allows it to return to its original shape. If you have several of the same bra, try hanging them in your closet on a belt or tie organizer. You can keep track by marking hooks for each day of the week. Or divide your lingerie drawer into two sections: one to "wear" and one to "air." If you own four to five everyday bras, wear them two to three times a week and wash them once a week—they could last up to a year.

4. **Be gentle.** Once you've made an investment in several nice bras, you'll want them to last as long as possible. Hand wash (or wash on gentle cycle in a mesh lingerie bag) with a mild detergent. Always air dry. Drying bras in the dryer will break down the fabric and wire, forcing you to replace them sooner.

CHAPTER THREE

Sprouting: From Buds to Blossoming Boobs

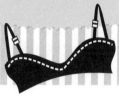

When I was about eight or nine, I was lying on the couch with my head on my mom's lap. She had her arm around me, and her hand on my chest. She kept moving her arm to a position where I couldn't breathe very well, so I kept moving her hand back so I would be comfortable. The last time she moved her hand away, I realized the reason she was moving it was that her hand was on my little boob. So, either I could have a hard time breathing and have my mom's arm around me, or move and not have her arm around me. I chose to choke.

—48C/D, AGE 27

I was really annoyed when I first got breasts. I was always playing "shirts and skins" with my brothers. Once I had boobs, I couldn't be a "skin" anymore. It seemed completely arbitrary and unfair.

—36B, AGE 44

Boobs change our lives. They don't necessarily make things better or worse, but they definitely force us to adjust to their arrival. And we don't get a lot of choice in the matter, either. Breast growth happens at its own pace, and on its time frame. Sometimes it can feel interminably slow, or be way too fast. It's not like having a period, either. Our boobs are out in front; they're subject to public observation and, at times, judgment. Sure, we can camouflage our natural shape under certain clothes, but we can't hide them all the time, especially in the girls' locker room. Then there are those pesky boys, always anxious to bring up the boob-growth topic as if it were some all-school matter of interest. Finally, we may have Mom, Dad, siblings, or extended family compelled to weigh in with their opinions. There could be some days we wish the whole business hadn't erupted on our chests. But there's no turning back the biological clock, so we'd better learn how best to live with our new bosom buds.

BREAST EXPECTATIONS

While media reports suggest that girls, on average, are going through puberty younger than their mothers and grandmothers, scientists disagree whether that's really the case. According to Joan Jacobs Brumberg in *The Body Project,* girls in the nineteenth century didn't have their first period until fifteen or sixteen years old.[1] But menarche (your first period) is only one sign of early puberty, which also includes the development of breast buds and the appearance of pubic hair. In 1997, one study found that puberty was starting as young as eight in black girls and nine in white girls.[2] But those who start their period that young may reflect a very small percentage of the population.[3] Increased body mass index and obesity are two factors that have been suggested as possible causes of the earlier onset of menses, generally by six months to one year.[4] Environment and behavior definitely play a role when it comes to your body clock, whether it's weight gain at an early age or better nutrition that's resulting in physical changes.

In cultures with more disease and malnutrition, girls menstruate at a later age and less often.[5] Today, a young girl may physically look like a grown woman, but she might not possess the emotional or psychological maturity to handle such transformations. How she feels about her boobs can play a big part in how she feels about herself.

Getting boobs is good news for most girls. Some believe that if you start looking more like a grownup, you might be treated with more respect and less like a little girl. Maybe you hope that parents, teachers, and others will start paying attention to your opinions and ideas. But when you're in the midst of all those hormone-induced physical changes, it can often feel like you're stuck in some strange dream. You wonder if you'll ever get back to feeling like your old self again. Going through puberty, while full of expectation, can also be pretty annoying. And when it comes to our breasts, it can also be very surprising. "Girls approach development in one of two different ways," says Marja Brandon, a sex educator and head of Seattle Girls' School. "They're either terrified of it and don't want it to happen, or they can't wait—and most of the time they have both feelings simultaneously."[6] It can be scary because people start reacting differently to how you look on the outside while you're still the same girl on the inside.

You need to get ready to expect the unexpected. Breast growth is unique to each girl and often varies even between your own two breasts. Plus, a girl's hormonal adventure begins years before our opposite sex counterparts have a clue as to what lies ahead. The average age for the onset of puberty in girls is age ten, compared to twelve for boys. And what's the biggest fallout from this jump start? As young women, we must physically adjust to new and often rapid changes to our blossoming bodies—plus cope with less-mature males' awareness of our newly maturing self. The only consoling fact you might keep in mind is that boys at this age are just as worried about penis growth and size as you're concerned about your developing breasts.[7]

As it turns out, we're probably our own worst boob critics during

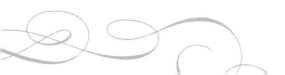

this time. According to a body image poll by *Psychology Today,* 54 percent of girls between the ages of thirteen and nineteen are dissatisfied with their appearance.[8] Comments that focus attention on our body parts can create anxiety and even greater self-consciousness. Any remark, whether made in sympathy, praise, or as a joke, can be misunderstood. Parents, relatives, and our very own girlfriends (boob-developing sisters, no less) can say and do things that leave lasting and sometimes devastating impressions on our psyches. And it's not just what we hear that changes our self-image. It's also what we see. Data compiled from twenty-five separate studies shows that young girls exposed to pictures of the thin, idealized media body type feel more depressed and angry, and have more body dissatisfaction, than girls who have viewed images of average-size models or inanimate objects.[9] As we learned in Chapter 1, only 1 percent of the population possesses a body similar to those digitally enhanced and airbrushed female images we see in the media. There's no reason to compare yourself to a likeness that even the model in the photo can't attain. Rather than fixating on this unachievable ideal, let's look at how real girls grow into their real, womanly breasts.

A GIRLS' PRIMER

The rate at which breasts grow varies greatly from girl to girl; some start off very "flat-chested" and end up with large breasts; others have large breasts at an early age. Often one breast grows more quickly than the other.
—Dr. Susan M. Love[10]

A great way to address our potential anxieties is to get the true boob scoop. Physicians separate breast development into five distinct stages (see diagram).[11] Not everyone goes through each one of these stages, nor do we experience them for the same length of time. Some of us may skip one phase, speed through others, or take what seems like forever to reach full growth. Blossoming bosoms proceed at their own individual pace!

HOW LONG DOES IT TAKE?

Stage 1 starts when you are still a child. The areola is flat and only the nipple is raised.

Stage 2 can begin as early as seven or eight years old or as late as fourteen. A small "breast bud," made up of fat, milk glands, and tissue, begins to form under the nipple. The areola grows wider and larger, and the nipple becomes raised. This stage can last for a few months or a couple of years or more.

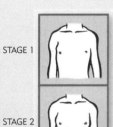

STAGE 1

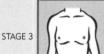

STAGE 2

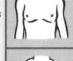

STAGE 3

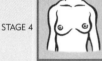

STAGE 4

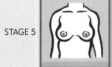

STAGE 5

THE FIVE STAGES OF BREAST DEVELOPMENT

Stage 3 is more of the same process, but the areola continues to grow. The breast tissue increases, and you start to look as if you have breasts. They may be more pointed at this stage, and they're not the final form you'll have as an adult woman. This is usually the time when girls start thinking about buying a bra.

In **Stage 4**, the areola and nipple come together to form a "mound" on your breast. Many girls skip this stage. By **Stage 5**, you have fully formed breasts.

During all of these stages, you may experience pain, itching, and tenderness, especially once your period begins. Often, one breast will grow at a different rate than another, or feel sore or a bit lumpier. The entire process could take just a few months or up to ten years. Most girls, though, will complete development in four to five years.

Whatever the outcome, and however long it takes to reach that magical fifth stage, you'll be the proud owner of a unique pair of breasts. As you're developing, you may find it helpful to compare yourself to photos of other real (nonairbrushed) breasts. That way you'll get a good view of the boob-spectrum. (Check out the Boobliography in the appendix for some helpful resources.) You're guaranteed to never see another set quite like your own.

Tabitha Lahr

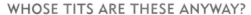

WHOSE TITS ARE THESE ANYWAY?

I was the same size in grade seven as I am now.
This is very different from my mother, who is huge, and she kept
promising that I would inherit her breasts; however, they have
yet to appear, and at twenty-eight I'm losing hope.

—32A, AGE 28

You may be puzzled if your breasts don't resemble those of other female family members, especially your mother's. But remember that your genes come from both sides of the family. Since breasts are mostly made of fat, you inherited the way it's distributed on your body from one or both of your parents. Maybe the women from your dad's side of the family more closely resemble your body type. Maybe you owe your size and shape to some other distant relative. There's no exact science when it comes to breast inheritance.

Breasts can also differ from what is thought to be the ethnic expectation of "normal." Sharon, a Japanese American woman, grew into a 34DD, while her mother and other Japanese American girl-friends possessed culturally expected smaller breasts. "I developed early, and since my mother didn't talk about anything sexual or about the body, I felt isolated. I felt boys were looking at them like they were an oddity." Sharon felt awkward not just when comparing herself to her mom but also in relation to her entire culture. It's easy to define "different" in negative terms, but no two breasts are similar, so we might as well enjoy and celebrate our own diversity.

Then again, we may turn out just like mom or sis and still feel strange. Some young girls are mortified to think they might have breasts as large (or as small) as those of a female relative. You might like all those references to looking just like pretty Aunt Helen, and you might admire her taste or style, but that doesn't mean you'll be as comfortable as she is with the same-size boobs.

Maria spent her formative years trying to hide what to her were painful and uncomfortably large DDD breasts for her five-foot frame. "My mother, on the other hand, loved her breasts, and flaunted them by wearing plunging necklines. She tried to be nice taking me bra shopping, but it was hard for her to be empathetic when she couldn't relate to my distress." Maria finally chose to have her breasts surgically reduced later in life. (For more about breast surgery, see Chapter 11: Cut and Paste.)

BUMPS, LUMPS, HAIRS (AND OTHER CURIOUS STUFF)

When the breast bud first appears in Stage 1, you might feel it as a lump below the nipple. This is fairly common and isn't anything to worry about.[12] Breast cancer in teens is a very rare occurrence, and only 10 to 15 percent of all breast cancers are diagnosed in women under the age of forty. (For more information on breast cancer, see Chapter 10: In Sickness and in Health.) In the sometimes lengthy process of getting our full boob growth, we may experience different sensations, such as lumpiness, pain, itchiness, soreness, or swelling.

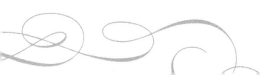

In rare cases, some lumps are really extra nipples. They are found along the milk ridge and often occur in women whose mothers have or had extra nipples. They may look more like a mole than a nipple and are nothing to worry about. Boys can have extra nipples, too. Model and actor Mark Wahlberg once thought about having his extra nipple removed but now says, "I've come to embrace it. That thing's my prized possession."[13]

Here's a list of other, more common concerns:

BUMPS AND LUMPS

Some of us have a few or many bumps on our areolae. These are perfectly normal. Known as Montgomery's glands, they lubricate the nipple area when our boobs are enlisted in the job of nursing a baby. Just before or during your period, you might also find other lumps and bumps under your armpits. These often go away within the week. Some breasts just seem lumpier than others, so it's good to get to know your girls and what's normal for your body. If you have any concerns at all, don't hesitate to see a nurse practitioner or doctor.

Some girls and women with numerous lumps are diagnosed as having fibrocystic disease. But according to Dr. Susan Love, there is no such thing. "'Fibrocystic disease' is a meaningless umbrella term—a wastebasket into which doctors throw every breast problem that isn't cancerous. The symptoms it encompasses are so varied and so unrelated to each other that the term is wholly without meaning."[14] Scientists now believe that it's more useful to talk about lumpy breasts as going through "fibrocystic changes." It's a condition, rather than a disease, and one that affects half of all women at some point in their lives.[15] (For further discussion about benign, or noncancerous, breast conditions, see Chapter 10: In Sickness and in Health.)

HAIRS

Nipple hair is normal. Some of us have one or two strands, others have more. If they bug you, there are safe ways to remove them.

STRETCH MARKS

Some girls' boobs grow so rapidly that their skin literally can't keep up with such fast progress. If that should happen to you, you may be left with stretch marks. Some start out red, but often fade to white. If they bother you, there are ways to make them less noticeable.

DISCHARGE

You might find your nipples secreting a clear white or yellowish fluid at certain times of the month. This, too, is normal; it's your body's way of keeping multiple nipple ducts open.[16] If this is happening with only one breast, doesn't go away in a few days or a week, or changes in color or contains blood, check with a physician.

INSIDE-OUT NIPS

Nipples come in every dimension, including flat and inverted (turned inward). Sometimes you outgrow this condition, but even if you don't, it won't stop you from breastfeeding. You can also reverse inverted nipples with surgery, although it's not always successful and may interfere with future breastfeeding ability.[17]

BOOBS OF VARYING DIMENSIONS

Every woman has one breast smaller or larger than the other. This is known as breast asymmetry. Some women's breasts differ greatly, often up to one cup size or more, which makes it tough to shop for bras or fit into a bathing suit. Lingerie manufacturers have come up with ingenious and natural-looking ways to make two different breasts appear more even. You should consult with an experienced bra fitter or check out some of the web and written resources listed

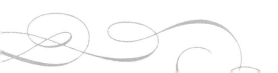

in the Boobliography. In extreme cases of breast asymmetry, plastic surgery is also an option (see Chapter 11: Cut and Paste).

PAIN AND SORENESS

Growing breasts hurt, and that pain is not always the same for everyone. Your breasts will also be more swollen and tender right before your period. Certain foods, such as caffeine, alcohol, or salt, may make matters worse if you retain water easily, so you might consider changing your diet for possible pain relief. But if you experience any pain that lasts for more than a couple of weeks, is worse in one breast than the other, or that makes you anxious or worried, talk with a nurse or physician to find out if there could be another medical cause.

RUDE DUDES, BAD BOYZ, AND MEAN GIRLS

The most painful thing girls may endure during their adolescent years is the taunting and teasing with regard to our breasts—from boys *and* girls. These breast bullies may be acting out their own body insecurities, but that doesn't make their remarks any less stinging or easier to tolerate. "At school, boys would tease all the girls with no or small breasts and make us feel inadequate. One particular boy would thump the girls on their breasts because he thought it was amusing," remembers Lisa, a 34A. Bigger-bosomed gals suffered other humiliations. "I remember sitting in math class and the boys were coming up to me with a ruler and trying to measure them. I was mortified! I started to walk with my shoulders slumped because I felt like it made them look smaller," recalls another girl, who's now a 34D. All girls, whether developing early or late, can be potential targets. Cathy, also a 34D, blossomed early, in fifth grade, and "was extremely self-conscious because all the other girls made fun of me." Many late bloomers feel thankful they didn't get their full growth until much later. One 34A (now a 36C) says, "My girlfriends always talked behind the backs of girls who were bigger. That made me glad mine weren't so big."

BARBIE'S BOOBY TRAP

Barbie was created in 1959 by Mattel cofounder Ruth Handler, who thought up the idea while watching her own daughter, Barbie, playing dress-up with paper dolls. She figured there was a market for a three-dimensional plastic playmate with a flair for fashion. Since that time, it's estimated that more than one billion Barbie dolls have been sold worldwide, and she's still Mattel's best-selling product.[18] The average American girl gets her first Barbie by the time she's three years old and collects seven during her childhood.[19] Many people criticize the doll's unrealistic body proportions, and studies have shown that it fosters negative body image in very young girls.[20] Ruth Handler, in her biography, defended Barbie's exaggerated dimensions as necessary to have the miniature doll clothes hang properly. Otherwise, Barbie wouldn't serve as a fashionable dress-up playmate.

Ironically, it has been estimated that if Barbie's original body dimensions were translated into a real woman's figure, she would measure 39–18–33.[21] Even Pamela Anderson's bodacious body doesn't stack up at 36–22–34. In comparison, the average woman measures 36–29–39 and weighs 143 pounds.[22] Any woman with a figure even remotely resembling Barbie's would be hard pressed to find fashionable clothes to fit her freakish dimensions, not to mention outfitting her size 3 feet.

In 1970, Handler was diagnosed with breast cancer and underwent a mastectomy. She soon discovered how difficult it was to find realistic-looking breast prostheses and founded her own company, Nearly Me, to meet this need. Handler died in 2002 at age eighty-five.

We should remember that this kind of verbal cruelty can have lasting consequences. And if such offensive remarks are directed at us, take heart that these perpetrators are probably more worried about how they look to us than how we look to them.

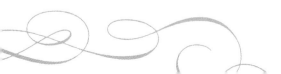

BRA BASICS FOR BUDDING BOSOMS

How can you feel comfortable when your body isn't? Some think it's by wearing a bra. Others think just the opposite. The question is not whether you should wear a bra, but whether *you* want to wear one. If it makes you feel better to buy one, go ahead. There are some days you'll want to wear it, and others when you'll cringe at the thought. This is a time of transition, of you getting used to your new body. You get to decide, although your family is probably footing the bra bill.

WHO'S TRAINING WHOM?

Until the 1950s, most adolescent girls didn't wear training bras. They existed, and had been available since the 1920s and 1930s,[25] but most young girls wore camisolelike undergarments until they had enough breast tissue to really fill out a bra. According to Joan Jacobs Brumberg, physicians and bra manufacturers began to tout the health benefits of wearing bras in the late 1950s. These miracle mound shapers were advertised as helping young girls grow into successful breast-feeding moms. "An adolescent girl needed a bra in order to prevent sagging breasts, stretched blood vessels, and poor circulation, all of which would create problems in nursing her future children," writes Brumberg.[26] We now know that bra wearing has no medical benefits whatsoever. There are even anti-bra groups that claim bras can cause breast cancer. In today's market, there doesn't seem to be a need to assign this separate "training" distinction to bras for smaller busts. Camisoles with shelf bras and one-piece sports bras fill in the gap nicely. Women may be fully trained in the importance of wearing bras, but due to a lack of manufacturing standards, we still need guidance on how to buy one that fits us well.

THEY'RE MY BOOBS, THANK YOU

Whether you choose to get a bra at the first sign of a breast bud or later, it's up to you. Parents seem to be the ones to notice our boobs first, and they might suggest a first bra-shopping expedition. One young girl who didn't want to buy a bra finally gave in when her dad said, "Okay, then I'll wear one, too." The thought of him trying to put on a woman's bra made her laugh so hard, she agreed to go out and buy one that day. Other girls hate the thought of anything tight across their chest and might feel better wearing looser-fitting camisoles, many of which have built-in bras. Finally, there's also the choice of stick-on bras, which have no straps or hooks and come in lots of fun colors. They're perfect for someone with smaller, just-growing breasts who doesn't want the hassle of dealing with conventional bras (see the Boobliography in the appendix).

If you've flipped through Chapter 2, you know there's plenty to choose from in Bra-la Land. And although there's no medical reason to wear a bra, many of us feel more comfortable when our boobs aren't bouncing all over the place. If you find yourself in that category, the first thing you need to do is consult with a professional bra fitter. How do you find one? Most high-end department stores or boutique lingerie stores employ trained fitters. Most of them are women, but in

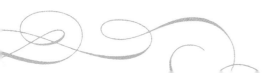

some places (particularly foreign countries), you might be surprised to find male fitters, too. You want to work with someone who has seen a *ton* of boobs—of all shapes, sizes, and dimensions—so choose experience over someone with little boob knowledge. She'll measure you and bring you lots of different bras in different sizes to try. (Don't worry, most bra fitters have you put on the bra with your back facing them, so you can still retain your modesty if you're worried about that.) Choose a bra made of a soft material, such as cotton, since you don't want to make your sore or tender breasts any more uncomfortable. If you're athletic and participate in sports, you'll definitely want to buy a couple of sports bras to keep your breasts secured (see Chapter 6: Mammaries in Motion). You'll also want to buy at least two bras in your size, but not many more. Remember, you're a growing girl (and your girls will continue to grow), so expect to go back for another fitting in the next six to twelve months.

If you're battling with your mom, dad, or other caregiver over how best to dress your girls, share with them the following possible solution to both your problems.

THEY'RE MY DAUGHTER'S BOOBS, THANK YOU

You may feel your daughter "needs" to wear a bra, but she may be resisting or is a bit shy about the process. Or she may come to you begging to have you take her bra shopping, but you're not sure if she's ready. How do you turn what could be a potential struggle into a win-win situation? Get her off to the breast bra-buying start! Make it a special "girls only" shopping day. You can drop her off in the lingerie department or other specialty foundation boutique. (Be conscious of the possibility that she doesn't want you there.) Make sure you choose a store that has experienced personnel and a wide range of merchandise. Leave her to get her girls properly fitted by the professional. Then pick her up when she's all done and celebrate a very uplifting day with a girls' lunch out!

GETTING TO KNOW YOUR NEW GIRLS

While teen breast cancer is very rare, that doesn't mean you shouldn't learn the lay of your mammary glands. Feeling your breasts once a month gets you used to what's normal for you. If you have some bumpy terrain (most likely during puberty), you can keep track of your topography with your own Boob Log, found in the appendix (p. 237). When you go in for a yearly physical exam, your doctor will perform a breast exam as part of that process. If you know your own breasts well, it will make it much easier for you to talk with your physician about anything he or she (or you) might find unusual. Because mammography screening is currently less effective on younger women, due to their dense breast tissue that's more difficult to read on film, it's unlikely you'll undergo that procedure. Once you turn forty, experts agree that you should have a yearly mammogram. If you've a family history of breast cancer, you may be asked to undergo screening at an earlier age. For additional information on taking care of your breast health, please see Chapter 9: Your Breast Potential. But if there's anything that worries or concerns you about your breasts, don't hesitate to ask your doctor or other health-care provider.

ODD GIRLS OUT

Can you change the size of your mammary inheritance? Yes. You can look bigger or smaller depending on the bra you wear; or you can correct an imbalance with many of the breast-enhancing inserts now on the market (see Chapter 2). There are also pills, lotions, and potions that might promise to change the size of your breasts, but there's no scientific evidence that they work. There is at least one breast-enhancing product (Brava) that some have found helpful, although it may be more work than it's worth (see Chapter 9: Your Breast Potential). Because your breasts aren't made of muscle, there aren't any exercises you can do to build up the breast tissue, although you can build up the pectoral

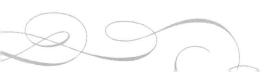

muscles on which they rest. If you gain or lose weight, either by diet and/or exercise, your breast size will shift, too.

You can alter your breasts through surgery, with implants, a reduction, or a breast lift (see Chapter 11). These are all serious and expensive procedures and not normally covered by insurance. Unless you have some congenital deformity, most reputable plastic surgeons won't perform breast reductions or breast augmentations on patients under the age of eighteen. Until that time, you're not fully developed. Since breasts keep growing into your twenties and even thirties, it's a good idea to be patient with your body. But in a few, rare cases (like severe asymmetry), it might be your only choice. Even though boys often outgrow the condition of gynecomastia (when boys grow breasts), nearly fourteen thousand cosmetic breast reductions were performed on boys under nineteen in the United States in 2006. Approximately nine thousand girls under nineteen had breast augmentations (about 3 percent of all such procedures performed) that same year.

CHAPTER FOUR

Talkin' Tits:
The Language of
Breast Size

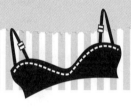

My best friend has huge breasts, so we are polar opposites in that respect. We both complain about our breasts . . . but for very different reasons.
—34AA, AGE 22

People think they know something about you that they really don't. If you are short and small breasted, they think you are "sporty." If you are big, you are a "slut."
—36C, AGE 35

We know stereotypes exist, yet who wants to be labeled based solely on outward appearance? We prefer to be appreciated for who we are on the inside. You've probably laughed at the occasional dumb-blond joke and other jokes based on stereotypes. And though one physical characteristic should not have the power to determine our lot in life, our wonderful breasts can sometimes define us. No woman consciously chooses her biologically determined breast shape and size (although she might try to change her silhouette with the help of a bra or some cosmetic procedure). We have what we have, and how we're treated because of that can have a huge impact on our self-image.

Women are criticized, or applauded, for how much of their breast shelf they reveal. In certain situations, judgments are made if we expose too much cleavage or wear too-tight clothing. We are often viewed as flaunting our sexuality (or "assets"), whether we do so intentionally or not. Because of their erotic nature, it's uncomfortable when a complete stranger makes some random remark about our breasts. "Nice rack" carries more unsolicited intimacy than "nice six-pack." We might laugh such comments off and think of them as silly, but they can be destructive, and, in certain contexts, they can qualify as sexual harassment. And it's not always men who make crass or overtly obvious remarks regarding our breasts. Women can be our own worst critics and the best at trading cruel barbs when it comes to another gal's girls.

Assumptions made about us based on our breast size and shape may cut more to our core because they're directed at our womanhood and sexuality. Breasts have power, both to sustain our offspring and provide us pleasure. These pockets of fat and tissue are the "chosen ones" in a way. They are admired for their soft round features and sensitive nipples. But if females had evolved to sport exceptionally long earlobes as a means to feed their children, we'd all be wearing something binding the sides of our heads instead of our breasts. We may show off our boobs, or keep them more hidden. When we reveal them, we are wielding a degree of power. We allow others to look at them and enjoy their beauty with a hint of sexuality. When we choose to cover them, we are exerting our authority over who will or will not see them. It's our own personal decision, either way. Defining women solely based on breast appearance takes away our right to define our breasts for ourselves.

BOOB BRANDING

Research shows that women with large breasts are typed as incompetent, immoral, immodest, and not very smart. Small-breasted women, on the other hand, are seen as competent, intelligent, moral, polite, and modest.

—CAROLYN LATTEIER,

BREASTS: THE WOMEN'S PERSPECTIVE ON AN AMERICAN OBSESSION[1]

We've all heard the comments, whether in high school hallways, college dorm rooms, or in Internet chat rooms. Small boobs mean you're athletic and studious, while large boobs imply less intelligence and more sex appeal. Scientific studies confirm we women perpetuate those stereotypes, too. Research from 1998 shows that Caucasian and Asian American women find larger breast size to be associated with more positive attributes, such as being popular, sexually active, assertive, confident, and nurturing. Smaller breast size holds negative attributes, including being depressed and lonely, although smaller boobs are also associated with intelligence and athleticism.[2]

Extreme stereotypes exist on both ends of the spectrum, leaving one to wonder if there is a medium or "perfect" size with which women might be happy, at least for themselves. Researchers have found that females are more likely to see their bodies on a part-by-part basis. Smaller-busted women who may be happy with other parts of their body may dislike their breast size. Larger-busted women who are pleased with their boobs might be preoccupied with their weight. It could be that breasts always look better when they are sitting on someone else's chest.

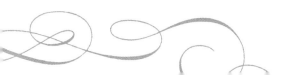

IDEAL VS. REAL PERCEPTIONS

*Men and women seem to assume that others' ideals are consistent with the
exaggerated, large sizes so prevalent in all forms of media. Individuals'
actual preferences, however, appear to be smaller and somewhat
more realistic than stereotypical conceptions of cultural ideals.*

—STACEY TANTLEFF-DUNN, *SEX ROLES: A JOURNAL OF RESEARCH*[3]

Perception seems to have little to do with reality when it comes to
boobs. "The few sociological studies that have been done about
breast size preference did not produce consistent results," says Caro-

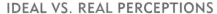

lyn Latteier in *Breasts: The Women's Perspective on an
American Obsession.*[4] Yet when women see larger
breasts on porn stars, or in men's magazines, we
assume it must be what men ideally hope for in a
female mate. Even when women rate their own
breasts, they often think theirs are smaller than
what most other men and women would desire.[5]

Scientists have tried to measure whether
males prefer larger breasts over other sizes, but such
studies have been contradictory and inconclusive.[6] Even when men
are found to prefer bigger bosoms, the size women think men prefer
is usually larger than what men actually favor. Flip those tit statistics
and guess what? Studies show that men believe women desire a larger
chest size in men than they actually do.[7]

A lot of these false assumptions are driven by society's mass marketing of a specific body type. Based on a study of the covers from the
four most popular magazines over the past twenty-five years, fashion
models' bodies have gotten taller and slimmer.[8] The average weight
and bust-to-hip measurement ratio of *Playboy* centerfolds has also
decreased over the past thirty years.[9] Flipping through *The Playmate
Book: Six Decades of Centerfolds,* by Gretchen Edgren, quickly confirms

SuzyLamont.com

these findings. You might also note that modern-day Playboy bunny breasts are higher, firmer, and more stacked onto their owners' torsos. These twenty-first-century boobs seem less soft and fleshy when compared to those of Marilyn Monroe and Jayne Mansfield from the '50s and '60s. That tits-on-a-stick look that's so popular today seems at odds with a typical female's curves. Indeed, the only time we appear to worship fat in our society is when it's placed over (or in some surgical instances, under) a woman's pectoral muscles.

bOObflash!

EXPANDING PECTORAL PICS

While female models keep getting taller and thinner, male models keep beefing up. A study of *Playgirl* centerfolds during the past twenty-five years shows that society's ideal male body is growing more muscular.[10]

These idealized breasts—round, high, and firm—have another thing in common: They remind us of our youth. Our culture values these young girls of yore for what they represent. In the evolutionary scheme of things, they are a signal of fertility, since they were apt to be located on the body of a postpubescent girl. Highlighting bigger breast proportions, though, speaks to the supersizing of everything in our society. Show a guy a picture of a steak. A bigger, thicker, juicier slice must be better, right? The gentleman in question may not even be hungry, but he's culturally conditioned to respond to adages that "bigger is better."

Advertisers are well aware that boobs have the power to grab and hold our attention. This is why they're used to sell everything—from beer to bookends. More than one restaurant chain has been founded

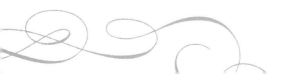

on the notion that breasts will get men in the door to buy burgers and chicken wings. Certainly, the Hooters brand is interested in selling you lots of other products. They have their own credit card, an airline(!), and the obligatory pinup-girl calendar. The bosoms on display in their advertisements and products are boringly similar to those seen in mainstream men's magazines. There is little variety shown in the packaging of boobs for mass-market consumption. But maybe that's the point. Give us all one simple, single image and there will be fewer individual breast tastes to meet.

If you take boobs off a glossy magazine page, though, and put them in an everyday setting, you may be surprised by the responses to real breast dimensions. In a study measuring men and women's perceptions of breast size (and whether they favored any specific size), students were asked to watch videos of an actress presenting identical material. The only major variation was the size of her breasts. When men viewed the videos, they rated the woman with medium-size breasts higher on both professional and social scales. Female viewers were not influenced by any particular breast size. It appears that males do, in some settings, think less positively of women with small *or* large breasts. The author of the study theorized that men may not be aware of their boob bias. Even more telling was how the actress responded to her own appearance as her breasts grew larger. She reported becoming increasingly self-conscious.[11]

GIRL GOSSIP

There's a sense that among women it's acceptable to tease or make critical comments about each other's breasts—especially large breasts, but we need to remember that our comments can be just as hurtful as catcalls from men.
—Meema Spadola, *Breasts: Our Most Public Private Parts*[12]

Women can be cruel to each other when it comes to breast size. Lisa, a voluptuous 36D, remembers how some of the girls on her high school swim team didn't like her because they said she always stuck out her boobs when she walked. Lisa was shocked and embarrassed when this got back to her from a couple of her friends on the team. "It was crazy. I wasn't aware of their power up until that point—that people could judge you based on the size of your boobs." Lisa recalls how her aunt had related a similar story, only hers happened in the workplace. One day she was called into a female supervisor's office, where she was berated for possessing such protruding body parts. She was asked to refrain from sticking out her 34DD breasts. Can you imagine the scenario if an employer asked you to quit sticking out your ears, nose, or big flat feet? Large-busted women may feel they have no choice but to hide behind baggy clothes or distort their posture by drawing their shoulders forward. Anything to deflect attention from their offensive orbs.

Consider Pamela Anderson, who was the poster child for breast augmentation several years ago. Late-night talk show hosts poked fun at her boobs, while tabloids made sure to show her breasts—fairly easy given her revealing wardrobe choices—from every possible angle. Her boobs were the butt of jokes, and she was often the first name used by anti-cosmetic-surgery activists when railing against our society's perceived fascination with bigger breasts. Why did we berate Ms. Anderson and not Dolly Parton? Equally large breasts are given different treatment when one pair is viewed as real and the other man-made.

Sarah Katherine Lewis, sex worker and author of *Indecent: How I Make It and Fake It as a Girl for Hire,* thinks "porn-size" boobs are "usually less about a particular aesthetic or male preference and more about availability: A woman with conspicuous breast implants is a woman who appears to have modified her body in order to accommodate male desire, whether or not this is actually the case."[13] Some women assume that women who get plastic surgery for bigger boobs do so solely for men's viewing pleasure rather than for the enjoyment of the wearer. But is this true? Many women claim that their reason for undergoing breast augmentation is about self-determination, and

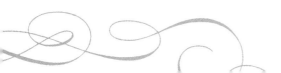

that it has nothing to do with pleasing someone else. Studies have concluded that such women are more motivated by their personal feelings about their breasts than by external opinions and ideals, such as a partner's unhappiness with their size or cultural ideals of breast beauty.[14] A 2003 study in the *Journal of Women's Health* compared women seeking augmentations with a group of physically similar women not interested in such surgeries. The group seeking breast enhancement surgery reported being more uncomfortable with their bodies, and many said they had been teased because of their appearance.[15]

There are some women who feel inadequate because they perceive their breasts to be too small. A woman with less breast tissue may feel disproportionate and less feminine. She may spend a lifetime wearing heavily padded bras or silicone cutlets and might ultimately choose breast enhancement surgery. (Breast implants are also used in conjunction with breast lifts and breast reconstruction after mastectomy. For more information, see Chapter 11: Cut and Paste.) Implants aren't an option for most women, however, either due to economic costs or physical risks. Experts disagree on the medical risks associated with augmentation, including the recent reintroduction of silicone implants onto the U.S. market. In 2006, augmentations outpaced liposuction procedures and became the number one cosmetic surgical procedure performed on women in the United States.[16] And with an FDA-approved silicone model now available, many assume that breast enhancement surgeries will only increase.

Our cultural obsession with figuring out whether a large-breasted woman has "fake" or natural breasts makes women even more self-conscious about their breasts. Women accused of being counterfeit when they've had large breasts for much of their adult lives might feel like they're being unfairly attacked. For some women it's a point of pride to have god-given big boobs, though not everyone can refute such speculation with a public sonogram—à la Tyra Banks. In her early twenties, Nancy was a 34B. In her thirties, her body shifted and she gained a few pounds. "I felt better with the extra weight," she says, "but people reacted to my bigger breasts with comments like: 'Did you get implants? What happened to your boobs?'"

Larger-breasted women seeking reduction surgery seem to get more empathy than those seeking boob enhancements—at least from other women. The choice to have a breast reduction usually stems from years of suffering from debilitating neck and back pain, not to mention the near impossibility of finding a bra that gives proper support. Seeking a surgical solution to alleviate pain and discomfort seems less frivolous and superficial than surgery that's considered wholly cosmetic. Breast reductions, like breast enhancements, ease negative feelings about body image. Women who have undergone breast reductions generally claim to feel better about themselves from having lessened their greater breast burden.[17]

LECHEROUS LOTHARIOS AND OTHER LOSERS

I had a boyfriend who was gorgeous but very immature and mean. One time he told me my breasts looked like marbles. Another time he said they looked like bananas. It took me years to get over those comments.
—34B, AGE 37

Women may be capable of "mean girl" comments that impact another girl's self-image, but it's men who do the majority of damage when it comes to our breast psyche. It can start at a very young age, too. Angela developed early and felt this brought her a lot of unwanted attention from boys her age, as well as from older men. "It made me feel self-conscious," she says. "I remember being twelve years old and a thirty-year-old man trying to pick me up in a subway." Or take the case of nineteen-year-old Marie, who says, "I've always had this thing in the back of my mind that my boobs aren't big enough. One time, my ex-boyfriend told me that the one thing he didn't like about my body were my breasts. Of course, this made me all the more self-conscious. Now

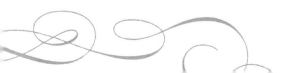

when I'm intimate with a man, I never want him to take off my bra."
It doesn't matter what your boobs look like or how comfortable you are with them when it comes to hurtful comments from someone whose opinion you value. It's important to remember that such remarks aren't really directed at us or at our boobs. They're made to make our abusers feel better about their own inadequate selves. They may well be envious or covetous of your gorgeous pair and only knock your knockers to make themselves feel better! Snide breast remarks are someone's way of trying to steal some of the power of your boobs. Don't let them. Remember that your girls are uniquely yours and are as special as their owner. If they (or you) are not appreciated, that doesn't mean you have to think less of them (or yourself).

Even when personal attacks on our breasts are not necessarily viewed as sexual harassment, they can elicit psychological wounds. It's not easy to ignore deliberate and often vicious verbal assaults on these symbols of our feminine self. Some of us don't let these boob-barbs get to us and just shake them off with ease. Others spend years trying to nurture their bruised breast selves back to better health. But there's hope for any woman who has had to put up with being teased or taunted. There are plenty of men and women out there who will love your one-pair-of-a-kind breasts for what they are: a special part of you. Read more about this in Chapter 8: Lovers Love 'Em.

RUDE REMARKS VS. DELIBERATE DISCRIMINATION

At work, men used to talk about my breasts with me in the room. I am a well-educated person, with degrees in art and anthropology, and an MBA, but I was treated less respectfully. Sexual harassment was not a term of the time, but today I could have sued the company and walked away a wealthy woman.
—36DD, AGE 46

If someone says something about your boobs, you might ignore it or simply blow off the message, along with the messenger. You might decide to tell the person that you don't appreciate their boob banter. But you could be offended, or even scared. Even if the person considers his or her behavior innocent, if those remarks make a reasonable person uncomfortable, they may be a form of sexual harassment. Whether it happens on the job, in the classroom, or while you're out in public, you should know what to do about it. Such comments don't have to be about your own breasts, either. Any behavior that happens in your presence and makes you uneasy or creates a hostile environment can qualify as harassment.

If sexual harassment happens in the workplace, you have certain rights and remedies under the law that should stop the harassing behavior from occurring again. If you are in a school setting, similar rules apply. Random remarks by some person on the street, unfortunately, don't qualify. They would have to rise to the level of physical assault in order to be deemed offensive, so in those instances you are better off ignoring the behavior. However, there are public situations when harassment laws can apply, such as when you're a guest or customer and you're mistreated by an employee of a particular establishment. But by and large, laws protecting women from sexual harassment apply to work or classroom settings.

There are no international standards for sexual harassment, and in some countries your only recourse is to contact a women's advocacy organization for guidance and support. But in the United States, personal comments about breasts can be deemed legally offensive. Sexual harassment was first defined in the United States in the 1970s and is considered a form of sex discrimination under Title VII of the 1964 Civil Rights Act.[18] The U.S. Equal Employment Opportunity Commission is charged with enforcing these guidelines in the workplace. Sexual harassment in schools, colleges, and universities is illegal under Title IX of the 1972 Education Act.

Sexual harassment knows no age limits. Girls and boys are often sexually harassed starting in elementary school. "Hostile Hallways,"

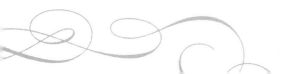

ON THE JOB: SEXUAL HARASSMENT DEFINED

Unwelcome sexual advances, requests for sexual favors, and other verbal or physical conduct of a sexual nature constitute sexual harassment when this conduct explicitly or implicitly affects an individual's employment, unreasonably interferes with an individual's work performance, or creates an intimidating, hostile, or offensive work environment.

Sexual harassment can occur in a variety of circumstances, including but not limited to the following:

- The victim as well as the harasser may be a woman or a man. The victim does not have to be of the opposite sex.

- The harasser can be the victim's supervisor, an agent of the employer, a supervisor in another area, a coworker, or a nonemployee.

- The victim does not have to be the person harassed but could be anyone affected by the offensive conduct.

- Unlawful sexual harassment may occur without economic injury to or discharge of the victim.

- The harasser's conduct must be unwelcome.

—U.S. EQUAL EMPLOYMENT OPPORTUNITY COMMISSION[19]

a study conducted in 2001 by the American Association of University Women, found that 83 percent of girls and 79 percent of boys reported being sexually harassed at school.[20] Although both boys and girls reported harassment (which included nonphysical harassment such as taunting, rumors, and jokes), the girls were generally more negatively affected by the conduct. They reported feeling less confident and more self-conscious and embarrassed than the boys, who were subjected to similar comments and/or actions. Girls often change their own behavior in response to these acts, choosing to avoid the perpetrator or participate less in class discussions. Nearly all the students claimed to know what harassment is, and many were aware that their schools had policies in place to deal with sexual harassment. More than half (54 percent) admitted that they had sexually harassed someone during their school years.

If childish teasing may seem innocent to one person, it might be felt or perceived in a different way by someone else. Girls' gossip or boys' suggestive remarks about someone's breasts can be offensive. And as studies show, such behavior hurts both the victim and the perpetrator. This is why educating children about sexual harassment early on is important. Teaching young children that their words have consequences will help reduce the incidence of sexually inappropriate comments and behavior.

The Internet, with its ease and anonymity, is another venue where harassment can take place. This can take the form of anything from unsolicited email porn-spam to more-harassing dialogue in a chat room or anonymous messages on a community networking site. Unfortunately, there are no laws that cover such unsolicited sexual remarks. And one out of five U.S. teens reports he or she has been sexually solicited over the Internet.[21] Organizations exist to provide tips and advice on how to handle cyber harassment. Some of these groups teach classes or provide educational materials for parents and children on how to stay safe on the Internet. (See the Boobliography in the appendix for a list of these groups and websites.)

STICKING UP FOR YOUR GIRLS

At work a guy came up to me and said, "Nice rack there."
It was uncalled for, out of place. I just rolled my eyes at
him, told him to get a life, and then ignored him.
—38C, AGE 28

If someone at work says something about your boobs that makes you uncomfortable, the first thing to do is tell the person that you

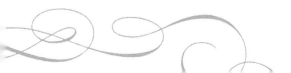

find his or her behavior offensive and ask them to stop. If they don't, then you'll need to consider taking further action. You can report him or her to your job supervisor or to your employer's human relations department. "Most companies have someone in charge of investigating these types of complaints," says Marcella Fleming-Reed, an attorney specializing in these kinds of cases. If your employer does not have someone who can handle these types of complaints, you can contact a women's support group or an attorney specializing in these types of cases. Once you take your problem to a supervisor, he or she is responsible for looking into the circumstances and asking the alleged offender for his or her side of the story. Many women fear retaliation in the workplace if their concerns are made public. The good news is that employers are exposed to legal liability if retaliation takes place. According to Fleming-Reed, "The Equal Employment Opportunity Committee ranks retaliation complaints a priority over discrimination investigations."[22]

The most important thing to remember is that any derogatory comments made about your breasts, or anyone else's, have nothing to do with you. Any type of harassing behavior is about exercising power over someone else. Women can harass men, too. Don't take these situations personally or think that you are somehow at fault. Your boobs are not the problem.

DON'T JUDGE A SET OF BOOBS TILL YOU'VE WALKED A MILE IN HER BRA

If each of us could trade places with a woman with bigger- or smaller-size boobs for a day, we'd probably gain a new appreciation for what we've got—and find that we like ourselves exactly the way we are.

To test this idea, Meema Spadola, author and producer of *Breasts: Our Most Public Private Parts,* spent a day wearing a bigger, silicone-filled bra. She had fun playing full-busted for a while, but she also discovered how much she didn't like the extra attention her plus-padded figure received. "Personally, I'm more at ease keeping my breasts out of the picture," says Spadola. "When I want to call attention to them, it's easy enough to put on a push-up bra and a low-cut blouse, but I can also hide them away. They're there, but they're not my central characteristic."[26]

Large-busted women don't have the luxury of taking off their boobs at the end of the day and putting them away in a drawer. They can't relate to the struggles of their smaller-chested sisters: an inability to create cleavage or feeling false or lost in a too-padded push-up

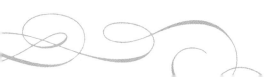

bra. Cheryl, who works to keep a low profile for her 32FFs, doesn't understand why men find any interest in her more-voluptuous size. "I know sometimes men have been intimidated by them, which infuriates me. What possible threat can large breasts be? It's not like a penis—what's it gonna do?"

EVERY BOOB HAS ITS PLACE

No matter what your size, you control the power of your boobs. What you can't control is when or whether others will apply some silly stereotype or judgment about you based on your boobs. Rather than dressing your girls in fear of judgment, you need to assess whether you want to create an environment in which your boobs are a focal point. It doesn't matter whether the setting is personal or professional; you need to check your mirror and make conscious choices about what makes your best-dressed shelf. To get on the track to self-managing your girls, consider the following steps:

Start with a proper foundation. The way your breasts appear to the world often has more to do with what you're *not* wearing under your clothes: the right-size bra. No matter how big or small, breasts change and bras wear out. If you haven't had a professional fitting in the past year, it's time to renew your boob wardrobe. A great minimizer bra will do wonders to keep big girls in place, while gel inserts and push-up bras can create the divine décolletage you'd like for a special night out. For more information on bras for your boobs, see Chapter 2: Bras: The Naked Truth.

Get real about your breasts. Take your breasts into account when choosing your wardrobe. If you've been picking out baggy clothes to camouflage your girls, you may be hiding features that deserve to be shown off. Include your breasts in defining the whole of whom you want to project to the world. In their book *What Not to Wear,* Trinny Woodall and Susannah Constantine list a set of fashion rules women can follow when it comes to their breasts: Big-boobed women are cautioned to never wear high, round necklines; the smaller-boobed among us should avoid scoop necklines. Their book features photos that flatter the figure while bringing attention to or deflecting attention away from particular breasts. The hosts of TLC's *What Not to Wear* program, Clinton Kelly and Stacy London, provide suggestions for every body type. Their book, *Dress Your Best,* lists style tips for work, evening, and even the weekend. Whatever your body and breast shape, there are plenty of options to choose from. Check out the Boobliography in the appendix for more books and style guides that give great tips for outfitting your girls from head to toe.

Harness the power of your boobs. Remember that you, and only you, have power over your own boobs. You may not control what others say about them, but you can decide what you want your breasts to say about you. Purposely revealing your breasts in snug clothing or a low-cut top will draw attention to your body and your sexuality. Are you uncomfortable in a too-tight sweater? Well, so are your girls. Does it make sense to wear a revealing top on a first date? It all depends on the impression you'd like to make (or the note on which you'd like the evening to begin). It can be fun to take your girls out in a flirty outfit, but make sure that you're wearing something up top that reflects who you are and not someone you think others want you to be.

People may use your breast influence as a weapon against you. You might dress very professionally on the job, but there's still some jerk who might make some snide remark about your rack. Consider taking action, or at least keeping a record of the offensive behavior. If such conduct continues, you may want to take your concerns to a superior or other employee representative.

Determine your breast self. Try not to internalize comments about your breasts. You live with your breasts every day, and you should learn to look at them from your own individual perspective. Like other parts of your body, they can have their good and bad days.

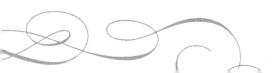

They're probably dissimilar to ones found in glossy fashion magazines. But those models are thinner, taller, and unlike 99 percent of the world's women. It's also possible that the images you see have been enhanced with the help of sophisticated computer software. Besides, you don't hug pictures in a magazine. You can't feel the warm softness of flesh against your body. Define your boobs for yourself, for what makes you comfortable in your own breast self.

CHAPTER FIVE

Unfettered Breasts: Exposing Your Girls

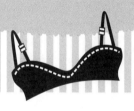

After hearing of topless beaches all my life, I must say it was more than a curiosity to me. However, after visiting one on a few occasions, I came to the conclusion that womens' breasts are just like any part of their anatomy; they're different from one another and come in all shapes and sizes.
—AMERICAN MALE, AGE 43

My friends and I used to drive up the Pacific Coast Highway in a convertible, wearing our bikinis, and we'd flip a nip to passing trucks. We were stone-cold sober. We just thought it was hysterical—and guess what, it was!!!
—36C, AGE 56

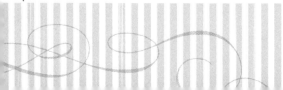

Undressing for bed at night is the equivalent of freedom for our girls. They're typically constrained for most of the day, and while letting them loose may be somewhat of a relief, it can still feel unusual, depending on what you wear to bed and whether you like to let them hang free. It's possible that the only people who have seen your breasts undressed are doctors, lovers, or someone who was inadvertently exposed—because of breastfeeding, or while at the gym. Maybe yours are the only naked boobs you've seen in person your entire life, despite the fact that naked breasts are put on display in our culture all over the place. Celebrity "nip slips," mainstream men's magazines, and PG-13 films are a few of the many avenues for viewing the naked female breast. It's a game of forbidden fruit (no boob pun implied) governed by an array of jumbled legal laws and often contradictory public opinion. A completely free breast may arouse as much suspicion as it does male sexual libido. Women have been accused of flaunting public morals, defying community standards, or creating a public nuisance for baring their breasts—even for breastfeeding. As boob owners, we all need to know what our rights are when it comes to our liberated breasts.

BARE BREAST DISTINCTIONS

Non-Western cultures have their own fetishes—small feet in China, the nape of the neck in Japan, the buttocks in Africa and the Caribbean. In each instance, the sexually charged body part . . . owes much of its fascination to full or partial concealment.

—Marilyn Yalom, A History of the Breast[1]

Can a woman legally bare her breasts in public? Yes, no, and maybe. It may seem odd that there are three different ways this question can be answered, but it all depends on who, where, and why you're flashing your boobs.

If you are a discreet nursing mother, you can breastfeed your baby almost anyplace in the world. If you visit a topless or clothing-optional

INANIMATE BREAST OBJECTS

Be they ancient sculptures, paintings of a nursing mother and child, or Renaissance celebrations of the female form, unfettered bosoms adorn the walls of our world's greatest museums. Not all represent the breast as nurturing or simply sensual. In 1830, French painter Eugène Delacroix immortalized a bare-breasted Liberty, her exposed bosom symbolizing defiance as she led her people to victory in the 1830 uprising after the French revolution.[2] By 1850, the bare-breasted "Marianne" became the emblem of the French Republic.

In the political realm, an exposed breast has stood for the qualities of virtue, solidarity, and survival. Another famously photographed half-exposed statue is that of the *Spirit of Justice*, located in the Great Hall of the Department of Justice in Washington, D.C. In 2002, then–Attorney General John Ashcroft's staff had her hidden behind $8,000 worth of blue drapes, claiming those made a better backdrop for press conferences.[3] Her boob wasn't put back on display until 2005, when Attorney General Alberto Gonzales's staff had the less-than-stylish curtains removed.

beach or other private swimming facility, you have the freedom to sun your girls in public. If you are a celebrity on the red carpet, or the victim of some unintentional "nip slip," your bare breast—with a requisite black bar or pixilated blur to cover the offending nipple—can be freely put on display in magazines, news shows, and across the Internet (often uncensored). If you're caught flashing your boobs in public, you may be arrested (although in the United States, a person snapping your pic won't be liable for reproducing and exhibiting that image). If you go top-free as a way to bring attention to some political cause, you may or may not find yourself in handcuffs. In most parts of the world, exotic and nude dancing is regulated in some way,

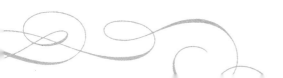

whether by physically restricting it through zoning, or by requiring the use of small pieces of fabric to cover up the one are(ol)a of a woman's breasts defined as posing a threat to public decency. These laws are typically enacted and enforced to protect those who might be offended by bare breasts, not the person baring them. Even in places where it's legal for a woman to bare her breasts, many women never take advantage of such freedom. This might be because they're too self-conscious or shy, or because they feel some shame about their bosoms. Yet in countries like Mali, where women walk around bare-breasted all day, boobs are no big deal. Breasts aren't even seen as objects of sexual desire or expression, only nature's milk machines.[4] In Western cultures like the United States, on the other hand, people have had to fight to push through legislation that protects a woman's right to nurse in public. It may be that in limiting our exposure to women's naked breasts, we've developed some mass amnesia about their original design and purpose.

THE RISE OF LACTIVISM

I am still pretty conservative about undressing in front of others, but when I was nursing my children, I did not care who saw what.

−36A, AGE 50

Women not only have the legal right, but a biological imperative, to breastfeed their children. Through the course of history, the popularity of breastfeeding has gone in and out of fashion. Wet nurses (women paid to nurse other, wealthier women's babies) were common during the eighteenth century, when it was thought that the upper classes need not bother with such lowly tasks. When baby formula arrived on the market, it was touted as a more nutritious (note manmade) and convenient replacement for mother's milk. But years of scientific study (see Chapter 7: Fully Employed Boobs) have proven that breastmilk really is best for baby. Today, pediatricians strongly encourage new mothers to breastfeed. And that's where agreement on this subject ends.

Everyone seems to have an opinion about the specifics of nursing a baby. Some object to any public feeding, others to those not done "discreetly" enough. Many people find a nursing mother a joy to behold—as long as the baby attached to her breast is a year old or younger. In other cultures, it's the norm for toddlers and beyond to nurse until they wean themselves. Here in the United States, moms have been charged with sexual abuse for breastfeeding older children or have lost custody of children because of extended breastfeeding. Numerous lactation activist groups have been formed not only to protect a woman's right to breastfeed but to protest any infringement of that right. This means they're involved with more than just providing women with advice on how to breastfeed successfully. Many groups are taking a stand and lobbying for laws to protect a woman's right to let her boobs function simply as nature intended.

Activism surrounding breastfeeding is a recent trend in the United States. La Leche League, now a worldwide organization supporting breastfeeding moms, was founded in 1956 when the boob-fed babe was completely out of fashion. Seven women joined forces to give this organization its start, and it now reaches women in thirty-four countries around the world.[5] But in the early 1990s, only five states had laws on their books pertaining to breastfeeding. Since that time, countless volunteer hours have been dedicated to ensure that public breastfeeding is specifically exempted from indecency laws, and other statutes are in place to protect nursing moms at work, in custody situations, or in any other number of ways.

Unfortunately, laws themselves do not change people's minds about whether a breast can be put on view, even for baby's sake. A 2001 national survey by the American Dietetic Association found that 43 percent of those polled believe women have the right to

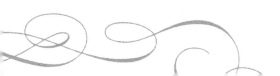

breastfeed in public places, but only 27 percent think it's appropriate to show a woman breastfeeding her baby on TV.[6] Another study that compared changing public attitudes about breastfeeding between 1999 and 2003 found fewer folks are comfortable when mothers breastfeed a baby near them (48 percent, down from nearly 50 percent in 1999); meanwhile, those who think mothers should only breastfeed in private places went up (from 34 percent in 1999 to 37 percent in 2003). Even more shocking is the increase in the number of respondents who believe that infant formula is as good as breastmilk, which rose from 14 percent to 25 percent in just several years.[7]

No one felt the impact of such attitudes more than Emily Gillette, who, in October 2006, was escorted off an airplane because she refused to use a blanket to cover her nursing baby's head. (This case was especially absurd since Gillette was seated at a window seat in the back of the plane, next to her husband, aboard a delayed flight. The flight attendant, the person ostensibly charged with keeping customers safe and content, found the breastfeeding activity "offensive.") After this incident, other mothers turned out in droves, staging "nurse-ins" at numerous airports in support of a woman's right to breastfeed her child—anywhere, anytime. But in Internet chat rooms, other women describe moms who nurse in public as "exhibitionists" and refer to breasts as "genitalia," the suggestion being that breasts have the power to procreate, not just lactate.

And it's not just real live nursing moms who make some Americans squeamish or uncomfortable. Even the photo of a baby at the breast on a magazine cover (no areola or nipple in sight) can result in hundreds of angry letters landing on the editor's desk. This is what happened in August 2006, when *Babytalk* magazine published such an image. Readers said they were "horrified," "offended," or feared their husband or young son might see the cover. What's fascinating is that it's not just men who may cringe at such images. Women were among the most vocal critics of the magazine's decision to run the image. Owning a set of boobs does not necessarily mean we all have the same breast view of the world.

UNDERSTAND THE BREASTFEEDING LAWS IN YOUR STATE

Most breastfeeding legislation in the United States is relatively new to our litigious society. Since 1994, when only five states had any laws pertaining to breastfeeding, thirty-nine have added some type of statute on the books either: (a) exempting nursing from public indecency laws, (b) protecting a woman's right to nurse her child in public, and/or (c) other legislation that can range from safeguarding nursing mothers in the workplace or prohibiting daycare facilities from discriminating against breastfed babies. But just because there are laws on the books in your state doesn't guarantee you'll be welcomed to nurse anywhere outside of the privacy of your home. According to Melissa R. Vance, author of *Breastfeeding Legislation in the United States,* "If a state does not have a law addressing public breastfeeding, it may mean that a private person, such as a restaurant owner, may have the right to ask a breastfeeding mother to leave. . . . Even where there are laws, there are still incidents where mothers are asked to leave or breastfeed their children in a public toilet facility."[8]

Other organizations, such as the National Alliance for Breastfeeding Advocacy and the United States Breastfeeding Committee, can keep you up to date on news and legal issues. If you feel you've been discriminated against for breastfeeding anywhere, please contact your local La Leche League or one of the above-named organizations for further information and support. For a list of helpful websites, see the Boobliography in the appendix.

BEACH BOOBS

I spent a summer in France when I was in my late thirties. One day I had time to kill on one of the islands off the Atlantic coast. I was sitting reading in the shade at the edge of the beach when the idea came to me that I could swim topless. I took off my bikini top and did the long walk down to the water. I was nervous at first—I'm pretty large breasted and always feel like I could lose ten pounds—but by the time I made it to the water, the self-consciousness was completely gone. I bathed for awhile, then made the long walk back, coming out of the sea like Venus. I noticed a young man looking at me with a sense of wonder. I'll never forget the look on his face. The whole thing made me feel completely amazing.

—34DD, AGE 42

The one place you will find women comfortably baring their breasts, or accepting of others doing the same thing, is at a topless beach. The former movie star Brigitte Bardot is often credited with starting the trend in the south of France back in the late 1950s. Seems she was one of the first to wear a "monokini" on the beach at Saint-Tropez. The monokini derived its name from the bikini, the assumption being that it was making reference to "two" separate pieces. In reality, the term "bikini" was taken from the site of U.S. nuclear tests at the Bikini Atoll in the Pacific Ocean, which happened the week before French designers unveiled their creation. The inference was that this new type of beachwear would have a similar explosive impact on the world.[9]

In countries such as Australia and New Zealand, it may be mostly younger women who venture out sans swimsuit tops. (One could argue that only the young have the time and leisure to hang out at the beach.) On European beaches, however, it doesn't matter what your age or body type. You'll see every kind of woman, from pre-sprouting to postmenopausal, going topless. And the women baring it all are unconscious of what others might think of their bodies. They are

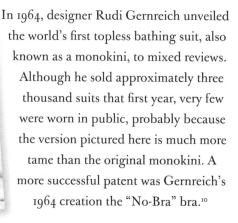

bOObflash!

WHATEVER HAPPENED TO THE TOPLESS BATHING SUIT?

In 1964, designer Rudi Gernreich unveiled the world's first topless bathing suit, also known as a monokini, to mixed reviews. Although he sold approximately three thousand suits that first year, very few were worn in public, probably because the version pictured here is much more tame than the original monokini. A more successful patent was Gernreich's 1964 creation the "No-Bra" bra.[10]

out enjoying the sun, sand, and surf. As one young twentysomething American girl said of her first bare-breasted experience on a beach in Italy: "I felt wonderful! There is nothing better than swimming in the beautiful blue-green Mediterranean sea with naked boobies."

Not all American women feel comfortable around such breast nudity. "I was too modest," says a mother of two girls, recounting her experience in the south of France. "I rely on my bathing suit top to give me the lift I've lost, so I wasn't about to let my boobs hang down and out." Others have similar stories—reacting to the various boobs on display not with sudden inspiration for their own unique beauty, but with fear their breasts might be viewed as unusual. A lifetime spent wearing bras that give women all a similar uplifted look can make it difficult for us to accept the fact that breast differences are

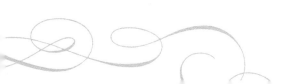

WORLD'S TOP TOPLESS BEACHES

Every year, *Forbes* reports on the best breast-baring beaches in the world. Many U.S.-run hotels can be found at these destinations, even though they are often legally restricted from offering these same topless bathing options at their own U.S. properties. In 2006, they were:

Anse du Gouverneur, St. Barts, French West Indies
Black's Beach, San Diego, California
Clifton Beach, Cape Town, South Africa
Copacabana Beach, Rio de Janeiro, Brazil
Illetes, Formentera, Spain
La Voile Rouge, Saint-Tropez, France
La Salinas, Ibiza, Spain
Manly Beach, Sydney, Australia
Nikki Beach, Saint-Tropez, France
Paradise Beach, Mykonos, Greece
Plage de Pampelonne, Saint-Tropez, France
Santa Maria, Forte Dei Marmi, Italy
South Beach, Miami, Florida[11]

anything but inequalities. Unlike men exposed to a variety of breast forms, many women cannot fathom such an appreciation for boob diversity. Which is too bad, because witnessing a plethora of ordinary bare breasts only confirms one truth: that few unclothed women possess the ideal breast featured in advertisements today.

Some Las Vegas, Nevada, resorts—intentionally catering to the young and uninhibited—have recently started offering "European-style sunbathing" at select swimming pools. This amenity is provided to guests at a sex-biased price. At Mandalay Bay's Moorea Beach, gentlemen pay $40-$50, while women are charged $10. The Mirage advertises its Bare pool (the "B" in this logo is missing its backbone, so there's no mistaking what's being "bared") at $30 for men and $10 for women. Other hotels bring the price down to as low as $20 for men—providing a more equal opportunity to witness ordinary, vacationing bosoms. Discriminatory pricing? At least it's cheaper than a plane ticket to the beaches of Europe, Australia, or the South Pacific.

In addition to topless beaches and private stateside pools, you can also bare more than just your breasts by joining a nudist or naturist club, which exist worldwide. Many such groups advertise themselves as "family friendly," although some have argued that these resorts are playgrounds for camera-toting pedophiles. To learn more about pro-nudity organizations, turn to the Boobliography.

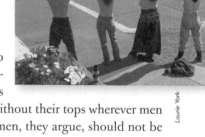

TOP-FREE PROTESTATIONS

The Top Free movement (so-called to distinguish itself from a less savory association with "topless" dancers) believes that women should be allowed to go without their tops wherever men are permitted that same freedom. Women, they argue, should not be discriminated against because their breasts have the ability to lactate. They feel that keeping women's bare breasts hidden causes them to be "objectified" as sexual objects, leads to sexual harassment, and lowers rates of breastfeeding, among other social ills.

In 1996, Ontario became the first Canadian province to become legally top-free, due to the success of a lawsuit filed by Gwen Jacob. Back on a hot summer day in 1991, then-nineteen-year-old Jacob removed her shirt and walked down a city street to protest laws that allowed males, but not females, the privilege to do so.[12] Her case was finally won on appeal on the grounds that by merely taking off her top,

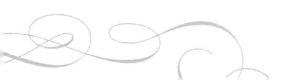

she did not violate community decency laws. As it turned out, it was the act of *not* doing something with her breasts that won her freedom.[13]

A similar conclusion was reached in the United States in 1992 when the New York Court of Appeals reversed the conviction of the Top Free 7, a group of seven women who dared to bare their breasts in public in 1986 and who were promptly arrested for their indiscretions. The court held that the statute under which the women were charged was related to lewd conduct, and in the absence of such behavior, the women were found innocent under that specific state statute. The aptly named Judge Titone concurred with the majority but opined that the state had "offered nothing to justify a law that discriminates against women by prohibiting them from removing their tops and exposing their bare chests in public as men are routinely permitted to do." He agreed with the Top Free 7 argument that such laws violated the women's equal protection rights.

Through the years, litigants have been successful in other provinces and states, but not everyone is interested in fighting a court battle to gain top-free rights. Canada is home to the Topfree Equal Rights Association (TERA), a group working since 1997 to defend women who have found themselves on the wrong side of the law when baring their breasts. Its helpful website recounts legal battles with indecency laws in Canada and the United States and includes such stories as the harassment of breastfeeding moms or the bizarre case of a sculptor commissioned to produce the figure of a mermaid without any nipples. TERA also attempts to provide information on various federal, state, and local laws, many of which have ruled that women can be top-free in certain instances, yet in other situations can still be considered criminal offenders.[14]

Since the 1970s, U.S. women have used their right to bare their breasts as a form of political protest. "Topless demonstrations became a means of calling attention to a wide range of women's issues, including pornography, sexism, healthcare, and safe sex," writes Marilyn

NIPPLES OF MASS DISTRACTION (NMDs)

Obscenity laws in the United States carefully regulate the exposure of both male and female genitals. But women are further restricted from showing that part of the breast below the top of the areola: our unique nipples. You can wear a skimpy tube top, barely there halter, or simply stick-on pasties—just as long as your nips are "covered," you're legal.

Many of these laws were written to regulate the billion-dollar adult industry. It was the owners of topless dancing establishments that fought the legal battles in the courts to ensure the right of their employees to exercise free expression under the First Amendment. But several courts, including the U.S. Supreme Court, have ruled that requiring G-strings and pasties does not infringe on any dancer's constitutional rights.

The irony, of course, is that pasties bring even more attention to the very part of the nearly nude female form that the law hopes to cover up: our nipples of mass distraction (NMDs). Hidden by a pair of twirling tassels, NMDs are even further eroticized. Many feminists argue that as long as women's bare breasts are forbidden from view, the adult industry will hold a monopoly on their indecent exposure. NMDs may, after all, be the most powerful (economic) weapon in U.S. history.

Yalom.[15] More recently, Breasts Not Bombs, a California grassroots coalition, has been staging topless protests to oppose the war in Iraq. Its message is that the war itself is indecent, not breasts.[16] In all of these situations, it's left up to local law officials to decide whether to make an arrest and prosecute the offenders. Public nudity is categorized as a public nuisance in many of these cases. If your boobs stop traffic, or create a commotion, you may just get a citation or find yourself in court. Each municipality, or other governing body, may have its own definition of what is acceptable unclothed conduct. If you decide to bare your breasts to make a political statement, it's wise to get to know the laws in your city, county or state.

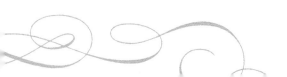

The Strong Breast Revolution isn't a real revolution; it's the name of a play, written by a Canadian playwright, and last staged to celebrate the 2003 Breast of Canada calendar. The play features actresses with their breasts bared and "deals with themes of breast cancer awareness, sexuality, breast feeding, adolescent body image, and even the fun of 'playing with your breasts.'"[17] Sue Richards, founder of the Breast of Canada calendar—a top-free pictorial to further breast health education—is another one of Canada's advocates for top freedom.

TERA serves as a resource to many individuals and organizations by advocating top freedom for women. Topfree.com is a U.S.-based organization that provides a forum for members to discuss where women can go top-free. If you'd like to bare more than just your breasts, visit the Trade Association for Nude Recreation or Naturist Action Committee websites.[18]

Other artists have gotten on the unfettered-boob bandwagon by baring them in print or on film and video. Back in 1979, Daphna Ayalah and Isaac Weinstock set out to photograph breasts of ordinary women. They found their project changed the lives of their subjects, in that it allowed participants to see numerous pictures of "plain Jane" boobs. Those who sat for these breast portraits revealed more than their breasts: They all had their own unique stories to share with the authors. Meema Spadola's 1996 HBO documentary, *Breasts,* featured such filmed interviews with twenty-two topless women, including one transsexual. In 2004, the film *Busting Out* chronicled our society's fascination with breasts. Filmmaker Kathy Kiefer's *Boobalogues* also includes stories about breastfeeding, augmentation, and cancer. Although the purpose of such artistic efforts is to counteract the association of breasts as merely sexual, these titles are classified as "adult" because they feature images of topless women. For a list of such boob-liberated resources, refer to the Boobliography.

NIP SLIPS

I was once waiting tables when my front-closure bra blew under the pressure. The clasp broke and my bra flung itself open with an audible snap as I was handing someone their marinated chicken. I was wearing a white shirt, so going braless was not an option. I had to wear an oversize sweatshirt the rest of the night, and I looked ridiculous.
—36C, AGE 34

Whether intentional or not, there do seem to be more "nip slips" than ever in the news. From Janet Jackson to Tara Reid, accidentally revealing your breasts feeds those hungry paparazzi anxious to catch the famous off guard. For us ordinary folk, these may turn out to be just a blooper or a most embarrassing moment. We can only hope that our anonymous actions won't be immortalized by some errant camera.

Across the Internet, and in many magazines, the bared nipple is newsworthy in and of itself. Surf the web and it won't take long to find the most obscure photo of a public figure photographed from afar, with a tiny peek of areola accidentally spilling out from her designer wear. Why all the fuss? Because these are the nips of the rich and famous, and their slip-ups should be viewed as embarrassing or humiliating. Consider the following famous celebrity boob blunders, which took me all of two minutes to find online:

- **April 12, 1995.** Drew Barrymore flashes her breasts to Dave on *The Late Show with David Letterman*.
- **September 9, 1999.** Lil' Kim wears a sparkling purple jumpsuit, exposing one pastie-dressed breast, at the 1999 MTV Video Music Awards.
- **February 1, 2004.** Janet Jackson's wardrobe malfunction occurs during the Super Bowl XXXVIII halftime show.
- **November 8, 2004.** Actress Tara Reid's recently surgically

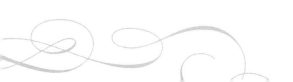

enhanced breast makes an unscheduled appearance in front of a horde of photographers.

- ➤ **May 14, 2006.** On the Cannes Film Festival red carpet, Bond-girl Sophie Marceau's dress strap falls and inadvertently exposes her breast to the quick-clicking camera crowd.

Each one of these attractive women sported a beautifully unique pair, including Tara Reid, complete with scars from her boob job. So why these incidents became front-page news in so many countries speaks to our breast-obsessed culture and the sexualization of the breast in the United States and beyond.

STOP NIP SLIPPAGE

There's more than one product on the market to help prevent unintended nip slips of any kind. You can try Hollywood Fashion Tape, adhesive tape sold in strips to help secure you in strapless or other revealing wear (including the ever-important wedding gown). The makers of the adhesive nipple concealers Low Beams also manufacture a latex-free medical-grade tape called Matchsticks. The double-stick strips come in a cute matchbook package. The great news about any of these products it that you can keep them in your purse and use them for just about any occasion: from a ripped hemline to a pesky sling-back that won't stay in place. See the Boobliography for more information.

SMALL-SCREEN BOOBS

Excluding pay-per-view porn, it's not unusual to see women's naked breasts on international television. The United States lags far behind other countries in permitting breast exposures on the small screen. Even during Janet Jackson's now infamous Super Bowl halftime flash dance, the thing most visible to the audience was the star-shaped nipple shield plastered on her semi-exposed breast. (This aspect of her wardrobe functioned nicely, thank you.) Other countries, such as those in Europe and Great Britain, regularly show adult programs or titillate audiences with completely bare breasts—whether it's to sell some product or as part of a humorous sketch. The U.S. Federal Communications Commissions—after the Super Bowl boob debacle—cracked down on some stations in order to ensure programming remain "family friendly" (although one wonders what could befriend a family more than a lactating nipple). Others argue that what offends our sensibilities more are tasteless but legal late-night visions of immature, black-barred bosoms, à la *Girls Gone Wild* commercials. But no one objects to paying a premium for cable TV featuring boob scenes from *Sex and the City*.

On stage, burlesque theater, has made a comeback complete with semi-dressed boobs, in the United States and other countries. Although originating as sketches performed at the end of minstrel shows, its more modern-day meaning is now almost synonymous with striptease. But that wasn't always the case. In its early years (1860s), burlesque shows were like a bawdy vaudeville, featuring a variety of comedic acts, parodies, and pretty women. One of the earliest acts from this time, Lydia Thompson and Her British Blondes, dared to bare their legs in (gasp!) only tights. This was during an era when long skirts covered most women's legs, so such revelations were considered scandalous but also served to make burlesque theater even more popular. Performers were masters of their crafts, with costumes and intricate acts geared to entertain the audience, à la Gypsy Rose Lee. By the end of its heyday, burlesque theaters had become all about the "tease" and pushing limits to get paying customers to attend shows. Before too long, women were gearing their acts toward stripping, revealing more flesh but less enthusiasm or creativity than their founding mothers (and fathers). By the early 1940s, burlesque was banned in many areas, including New York, where the original British Blondes had first landed in the United States.[19]

Today's burlesque performers say that the overexposure of the breast in soft- and hardcore pornography makes the art of tassel

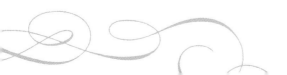

twirling quaint and conservative by comparison. "While live sex shows separate a woman's anatomy into distinct parts, burlesque celebrates the entire female form, in all its variations," says Ms. Indigo Blue, owner of Seattle's Academy of Burlesque.[20] The emphasis is still on the tease, but it's witty, playful, and sexy. Performers choreograph complex stripping routines to music and wear outrageous costumes and makeup, all intricately planned down to the final titacular twirl.

From small clubs to large venues, burlesque shows have gained in popularity. Rock star Marilyn Manson married (and recently divorced) burlesque artist Dita Von Teese, who was already famous in her own right. The annual Miss Exotic World Pageant in Las Vegas brings together more than one hundred international performers each year, and is sponsored by *BUST* magazine, among others.[21] The national Tease-O-Rama convention, founded in 2001, highlighted more than two hundred performers in 2005. It's not all about watching the professionals at work, either. Tease-O-Rama offers classes on the history of burlesque, tassel twirling, bra making, dance, and choreography—everything you need to know to get into the business of burlesque, or to just have fun in your own home.[22]

Ms. Indigo Blue teaches a three-hour tassel twirling class both in the United States and abroad. Anyone can sign up, and she's taught women of all ethnicities, backgrounds, ages, and sizes. Blue provides women with the basics of tassel design (what to look for in well-constructed pasties), how to properly apply and remove pasties, and how to get your ta-tas twirling. What she hears over and over again from participants is how much fun they have in these classes. "It allows us to play with our own bodies, totally in the context of silliness," says Blue. Women are given free rein to shake and wiggle a part of their bodies that is normally contained, constrained, and restrained. In this context, tassel twirling is a revolutionary act: a woman's breast as neither sexual nor nurturing, but fun and entertaining.

TAKE YOUR GIRLS OUT FOR A SPIN

Interested in the art of twirling? You don't need to attend a national burlesque show or live in Las Vegas. Many smaller communities feature burlesque revues, and national stars travel all over the country to hold workshops and classes. See what's available in your community, check out one of the shows, and decide for yourself. What you can expect is a room full of women of all shapes and sizes, in a decidedly unsexy atmosphere. Many classes include the tassel in the fee and provide instruction on how to place the pasties on your breasts—including alternatives for those with skin allergies to latex-based glue. There are various poses and postures, so just about anyone with any size breasts (even men) can learn to twirl.

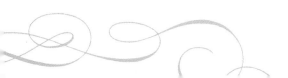

OVERT EXPOSURES

The creator of the *Girls Gone Wild* videos didn't invent the trend of women flashing their breasts at strangers; he just figured out a way to make money from their exuberance. Inspired by homemade videos of New Orleans revelers, Joe Francis founded Mantra Productions and his Girls Gone Wild empire. Francis and teams of GGW camera crews (only single, attractive men need apply) travel continually to spring break destinations, college campuses, or any other warm party-hardy spot where women might be induced to reveal their bodies. Francis captures young—eighteen- to twenty-five-year-old—uninhibited, and usually alcohol-imbibing females who are willing to flaunt their boobs and more. What do the girls get in return? Some the mere thrill, others a hope of rocketing to celebrity fame from such exposure. Usually all they go home with is a GGW T-shirt or cap and maybe some jeers and cheers from male bystanders. *Girls Gone Wild* video sales bring in some $40 million a year, with Francis reputed to have a $5 million yearly income. Women who have sued Mantra over the use of their images quickly discover it's actions are protected by the First Amendment. Lawyers have successfully argued that since the women are filmed in public places, Mantra is free to use their likeness. Francis and Mantra protect themselves by asking their unpaid talent to sign a legal waiver or model release form before the camera starts rolling.

According to Francis, the popularity of the Girls Gone Wild brand has changed the way women react to baring their bodies. He's been quoted as saying it "empowers" women. In 1998, when the business began, participants seemed more innocent and surprised by their impulsiveness. Today's GGW flashers appear to be more calculating exhibitionists, begging to be filmed in hopes of becoming a celebrity via Mantra's sales and marketing machine and late-night TV infomercials. The films have become more explicit, too. Simply flashing breasts is just a small part of what many young women willingly do.

Mantra's productions feature totally nude girls simulating sex acts alone or with each other. It's the equivalent of being a star in some low-budget porn film, minus the salary.

Francis hasn't limited his exploitation of the young and nubile to one sex only. Mantra now produces a *Guys Gone Wild* film series. But for whatever reason, the flashing formula is more financially successful when applied to bared boobs, not boys.

It's also no surprise that Mantra and Francis have been sued numerous times. And not just by regretful plaintiffs alleging they were filmed without permission. In a recent civil lawsuit, Francis was accused of gathering a group of underage girls at a hotel, plying them with alcohol, and offering them money to perform sex acts.[23]

BARED BOOB REALITIES

Just because we've got them doesn't mean we have to flaunt them. But we also shouldn't feel ashamed of our breasts. Breastfeeding is a wonderful gift to our children, and we have every right to stop and drop our tops for emergency feedings. If you prefer your modesty, then by all means, be discreet. But don't discourage other women who have chosen to breastfeed from doing so in public places. After all, the sight of a mom nursing might inspire another soon-to-be mom to give breastfeeding a try. If you see such a mom baring it all for her babe, give her a polite smile instead of turning away. (You can make a point of looking her in the eye instead of staring at her lactating breast.) If your boob should ever pop out impulsively, laugh it off. Remember that breasts are masses of jiggly and wiggly fun flesh (with one powerful NMD attached). Even the celebrities whose boob cameos were practically immortalized online have survived their boob faux pas, so some innocent exposure on your part is nothing to worry about. If you plan to bare your bosom deliberately, make sure you know what you're getting yourself into, or have the number of a good attorney on speed dial.

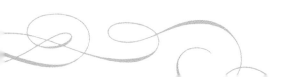

CHAPTER SIX

Mammaries in Motion: Life in the Athletic Lane

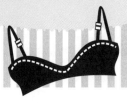

They don't get in the way, due to their size, and they're light enough to not need much support. So that's an advantage.
—34AA, AGE 25

My breasts get in the way all the time. I can't run, even strapped into the most structured sports bra. They still travel the opposite way [from] my torso and it's too uncomfortable. I also find it really hard to get a swimsuit to fit, and I'm too self-conscious in the pool or on the beach.
—32FF, AGE 31

The very existence of breasts on our chests is more apparent and sometimes problematic when it comes to participating in physical activities. We may not have thought much about them until we were forced, in some instances, to figure out a way to keep them out of the way. For some women more than others, this can be a constant struggle. Many of the more unusual breast tales revolve around our experiences on the athletic field or in the gym. Who doesn't have a humorous locker room story about boobs?

BOUNCING BOOBIES

My boobs were always in the way. When I was a cheerleader, they were bouncing more than the basketball on the court.

—38C+, AGE 50

Size definitely matters when it comes to participating in competitive sports. Smaller women may feel slightly superior in the athletic arena, since it's one place where they don't have to give their boobs much thought. Other women bemoan their larger and more cumbersome size, resigning themselves to wearing two—or three—sports bras to keep their girls strapped down. Larger-breasted women have also been known to wrap their girls in ace bandages or duct tape. Ouch.

As a competitive tennis player, Nicki didn't experience too much trouble with her B cups, but she does remember one instance in which they received a bit of a bashing. "One time my breasts were bruised because I was learning this new shot, and I guess I was hitting the boob in the same place every time I struck the ball. After five hundred times in a row, there was a mark to show for it." Janie found her smallish C cups "a tremendous advantage, especially in crew, running, and horseback riding. In fencing, though, I had to wear metal inserts in my bra," she says. The high seas were the ultimate challenge for another C cup: "The only time my breasts get in the way is when I'm sailing in dangerous waters and need to roll around on the boat. I actually have a scar on my right breast from scratching it on some rigging." Such injuries are probably more common than most people think. "Once in my karate class," recalls Kathy, a 38C, "I almost ripped my nipple off by hitting it with the tip of my *sai* [a dull-pointed short sword used in martial arts]. Aside from the pain I feel from bouncing, that's the first time they ever really got in the way." In some activities, even smallish- and medium-size women must acknowledge that all breasts have limits.

No one understands breast boundaries better than the female athlete who packs on a few extra pounds and finds it went right to her chest. One well-endowed 36DD "couldn't manage a backhand swing in tennis because my breasts got in the way." Roberta also found her 36D rack a challenge when swinging a racquet: "I finally realized my body needed to rotate along with my swing. In the beginning, my arm kept getting stuck on my boobs." Even less-than-rigorous activities can pose problems. Resa says her 36DD breasts make it "hard to do certain postures in yoga because they get in the way." And things can get even worse if your bra decides to be derelict in performing its much-relied-upon duties. "I played volleyball in high school," says one 42DDD woman, "and I was pretty used to them bouncing a lot by then. I recall a painful experience in practice once when my 'plastic' underwire snapped and it kept gouging me until I snuck off to tear it out. Then my one side sagged a bit the rest of the afternoon." New to the sport of climbing, Maria hasn't had too much of an issue with her 32FF breasts. "Although they can get in the way of the view when I'm trying to find my rope!" she said.

Bigger-bosomed women often don't worry about staying in a game that they've never been eager to join. Claudia gleefully recounts how her 32Hs got her out of high school P.E. "By high school, I opted not to participate in P.E. I was informed by the bureaucracy that P.E. was a requirement, at which point I instructed them to look at my boobs and then decide if I should really be doing jumping jacks with high school boys. Telling the principal to look at your gigantic jugs when you are fourteen years old is a real quick way of ending a discussion. I won." Others just take a more resigned approach. "As a full-figured woman, my breasts get in the way every time I get dressed," says 34DD Charmaine. "Clothes don't fit, and it's hard to do a chest press at the gym."

However, some women with abundant cups see their size as providing a competitive edge. One twenty-eight-year-old 38C soccer player thought hers were "great when I had to 'chest' the ball. It was awesome cushioning, and with a tight sports bra I became a mono-boob, providing a nice, squishy, even surface for deflecting the ball." Julie, a basketball player, felt her 36Ds "helped me defend the ball. I could use my hands to dribble and my breasts could assault the opponent, and I would rarely get called for a foul." Even if a woman doesn't find anything beneficial about playing sports with bigger breasts, she may learn that investing in the right equipment is the key to keeping her boob concerns to a minimum. As sixteen-year-old Vivian put it regarding her 32DD girls, "I do swimming, self-defense, lacrosse, tennis, hockey, and netball. I have invested a lot of money on good sports bras, and it has paid off."

NATURAL FLOTATION DEVICES

I don't think they really know how to make boobs stay in a good place in a bathing suit. Mine are always flopping around in there.

−36D, AGE 20

Our bosoms may seem to have a mind of their own, especially when we submerge them underwater. One woman snorkeling with her young children in Hawaii was puzzled by a group of young men who had stopped midswim to watch her and her family. Until she looked up and realized that her bathing suit top had come unfastened and was floating above her own head. A young girl's 34DDs made her think twice about her participation on her school's swim team. "During practice we wore two or three old suits for drag, and my boobs would get mashed down, and then during meets we wore really tight

SUPPORTING YOUR SISTERS IN STYLE

Not as pretty as their everyday half sisters, sports bras can often be more expensive (ranging from $45 to $75 and up). But most of us can't deny their comforting properties—and shouldn't spare the expense of keeping our own girls fit. Here's a short list of some of our tried-and-true bust friends:

B to C:	Donna Karan Soft-Cup Sports Bra
C to DD:	Donna Karan Active Sports Bra
C to DD:	Natori's High Impact Bra
Up to DDD:	Enell Sports Bra
Up to F:	Panache SuperBra High Impact Sports Bra

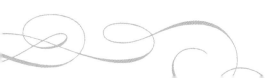

ones, so again, mashed down. Funny enough, this never seemed to stunt their growth. Or, oh God, maybe it did? And if I hadn't swum I'd have balloons on my chest. Wow. I've never been so grateful for swimming pools." But another gal had more trouble containing a set of smaller D breasts. "I distinctly remember one day at swim practice in high school I was wearing a black suit with turquoise stripes that was a little loose on me. I was diving off the block, and when I splashed into the water I realized that my left boob had come out of my suit mid-dive, in midair. When my head popped above water my coach said, 'Thanks for the show, but a little less skin next time.' It was mortifying." Investing in equipment to keep our girls well anchored ensures they don't take part in such escapades.

Lucky for the modern woman, swimsuit design has followed the same route as that found in bra manufacturing, offering a plethora of sizes and styles. You can order custom-made suits online, shop from a variety of catalogs (many of these retailers also offer sports and regular bras with similar sizing), visit a specialty swimwear shop, or choose from the selection available at your local department store. One designer, Malia Mills, has adopted "Love Thy Differences" as her trademark. Her company has engineered tops to fit different bra sizes and bottoms that consider divergent shapes. The idea is to celebrate the differences in all women by offering them more swimsuit choices. Sizes currently available range from 30A to 38DD and from 2 to 16.[5] No one store—or well-stocked website—can possibly meet the needs of the wide variety of body types found in nature. That's why it's important to approach the search for swimwear the same way you would to find a well-fitting bra. Take your time and be prepared to try on more than one style or size. Don't wait until a few days before summer or some tropical vacation to find the right suit.

If you know your true bust size, you'd be wise to preselect from brands available on the Internet. If you wear anything other than a generous B or slight C cup, you may be better off shopping online or at a specialty swim shop. There you'll find suits with different matching tops and bottoms, those with inserts or cutlets to accentuate your positives, and slimming lycra fabrics to hold in and support other parts of your anatomy. You may even find that having more choices leaves you less frustrated with the entire experience. Consider that Victoria's Secret, for instance, offers nothing larger than a D or DD cup top in their annual swimwear catalog. For women who are larger than that, it's not worth trying to squeeze your girls into a too-small size. Don't kid yourself. Swimwear is one area where you don't want to skimp on boob coverage. Given too little room, your girls could decide to follow the motion of the ocean rather than staying put in your suit. There are many online swimwear sites you can access, some of which are listed in the Boobliography in the appendix.

Just as there's a bra for every set of boobs, there's also a swimsuit out there waiting to turn you into a beach goddess. (Okay, that might sound like a stretch, but there's at least one that will provide you with the enthusiasm you need to go frolicking in the sand and surf.) The following are some flattering looks for accentuating or minimizing your breast assets. Larger-breasted women will want to focus more on support. Since boobs look best in balance to the rest of our bodies, consider the total package when trying on swimwear.

MAXI GIRLS

Underwire-bra-style bikinis
Solid colors or small prints
Wrap-front one-piece swimsuits
Halter style tops
Avoid strapless

MINI GIRLS

Halter bikinis with optional pads
Horizontal prints, textures, patterns
String bikinis (with ties to adjust)
V-neck one-piece suits, tankinis
Avoid strapless

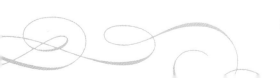

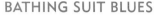

BATHING SUIT BLUES

When buying a swimsuit at any time, my breasts were never an issue.
It had more to do with my stomach and thighs, but that's another story.

—34D, AGE 47

"Ugh, swimsuits," is how one woman responded to the question of whether she felt limited in her choice of swimwear because of her DD breasts. A twenty-seven-year-old D cup complains that she "always hated choosing a bathing suit because the ones I could wear were always the old-lady suits. They had a uniboob pocket. I never felt like a girl, just an old woman." A voluptuous twenty-three-year-old bemoans how being a 36D means that "with swimsuits, there is never enough support and never enough coverage. Bikinis are sexy enough, and I don't need to have even more boob showing."

At the opposite end of the boob spectrum stand our A cup sisters, who have equally valid reasons to complain. "I can't wear a one-piece because they completely flatten me out," says one woman. Another notes how string bikinis are problematic because they cover the whole breast, "making me look even more ridiculously flat-chested." One woman said, "It's hard to find one that is flattering without it either sagging or being full of padding." And then there are the horror stories women recall about trying to supplement naturally smallish breast dimensions. Amy recounts the tale of a bathing suit she had as a teenager that was made for someone with cleavage, something neither she nor her best friend had at the time. "One day we came up with the brilliant idea to supplement our lack of endowment with puffs of toilet paper. We showed them off with pride. Unfortunately, when we decided to take a swim, gobs of toilet paper ended up floating in the pool."

Unlike bras, bathing suits are not just about boobs but the whole package. Regardless of body type, most women dislike swimsuit

RX FOR SWIMWEAR SHOPPING BLUES

- Go shopping at the beginning of the season, so you'll have more choices in styles and sizes.

- Check the calendar to make sure you're nowhere near your monthly menstrual cycle. (No use aggravating any potential PMS symptoms with shopping frustrations.) Also avoid any shopping outing after you've eaten a big meal.

- Enlist the help of trusted and similarly built breast friends. You can observe the advantages and disadvantages of certain styles on someone whose figure is more like your own.

- Choose flattering styles for your body type. If your breasts are the favorite part of your anatomy, play them up. If you have wonderfully long legs, work to highlight your great gams. Got a teensy waist? Show it off! It's not all about the boobs when it comes to feeling comfortable in the scant amount of coverage provided by today's fashionable swimwear.

- Avoid swimsuit catalogs filled with page after page of perfectly coifed, cloned body types. If it's too late, and you've already overexposed your powerful female psyche to such unrealistic images (remember: even the models don't look like their retouched photos), give yourself an immediate reality check. Go to the nearest swimming pool or beach and observe some real people without "perfect" physiques. It may even inspire you to temporarily put off your shopping expedition and just put on last year's suit so you can get busy having fun in the sun.

shopping. Which is why surveys have found that such purchases are rarely made on impulse (think shoes), and nearly half of us do it only once a year.[6] Another study shows that the act of trying on a swimsuit makes women more anxious and depressed and reduces our scores on math tests.[7] Whether you want to blame Madison Avenue's images of perfectly proportioned glamour gals or think this tendency rests in our female DNA, it seems that many of us may feel uncomfortable when it comes to wearing next to nothing in public spaces.

Another study found that flipping through catalogs, observing mannequins in windows of stores like Victoria's Secret, or glancing at magazines like the *Sports Illustrated* swimsuit edition can worsen any preexisting beef we have with our bodies.[8] Scientific experiments measuring a woman's mood after she's viewed a fashion magazine filled with digitally created thin models confirm we become more angry and upset with our own naturally unperfected bodies.[9]

Boobs are just one part of the equation when it comes to body image. So what do we really want in a bathing suit? According to an NPD Group survey, the majority of women ranked "fit" and "comfort" as the two most important qualities they look for in swimwear.[10] And to get the best fit for your tits, you may need to take advantage of those manufacturers catering to your unique needs. Clothing companies like Lands' End now offer specific swimwear features that target your self-described "anxiety zones." This allows you to choose styles and shapes that de-emphasize or enhance what you like best, including breasts.[11] For more information on swimwear websites, please see the Boobliography.

MASTER AND COMMANDER OF YOUR MAMMARIES

*My breasts are too small to get in the way; in fact I'm sure
I could jog forever with no bra and wouldn't feel a thing!*

—32A, AGE 28

"Your boobs should not stop you from playing sports," says Kate Starbird, a former professional basketball player with the WNBA. She once wore an undersized one-piece swimsuit underneath *two* sports bras just to play the game. And while there weren't a lot of large-breasted women on her team, she's known a few athletic women who lost a cup size or two when they took up the sport. Her sister, who was an avid soccer player throughout her youth, thought she lost her competitive edge at sixteen when she felt her boobs grew too big.[12]

While it seems obvious that wearing a sports bra would make participating in sports more problem-free, it's surprising how many women ignore this simple solution. When scientists measured levels of breast discomfort in women joggers, they found that more than half experienced pain.[13] Boobs don't just sway gently to and fro when we're running at a fast clip or even sprinting from the grocery store to the car. They lift up and slap back down on our chests. And the force generated by such rapid movements may result in our boobs exiting the limited confines of an everyday bra. Smaller-busted women probably consider themselves lucky enough to not have to deal with these

bOOb*flash!*

SPORTY BREASTS

Studies show that 56 percent of all women suffer
breast pain when jogging and often don't participate
in sports because of their breasts.[14]

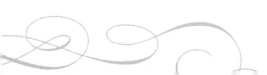

FROM JOCK STRAP TO JUG HOLDER:
THE BIRTH OF A SPORTS BRA

Some version of the sports bra has been around since the early 1900s.[15] But the most famous of its kind didn't arrive on the scene until 1977. It was then that three active women, Lisa Lindahl, Polly Smith, and Hinda Miller, got the idea to sew two jock straps together and market their invention as the Jogbra. They sold their company twelve years later to Playtex, and their design has continued to be improved upon and is now widely marketed as the Champion Jogbra. They are available in many styles and sizes, but thankfully none even remotely resemble a man's jockstrap.

problems. Even if it doesn't contribute to sagging, allowing our breasts to bounce all over the place can increase the amount of pain we experience when exercising. It's hard to imagine a man indulging in his daily athletic routine without encasing his own equally fragile precious pair in a jockstrap. We should strive to care for our own girls as well.

Shopping for a sports bra is a lot like stepping into some netherworld of action-figure enthusiasts. You'll hear words like "encapsulation" and "compression" bandied about, as if our boobs need to be tamed by mythical warriors such as "The Compressor" or "The Encapsulator." Active wear bras fall into two distinct categories: those that compress both breasts to keep them in place and those that encase each breast separately in a specific pocket of wire and fabric. The former gives us that "uniboob" look that so many women abhor, but it really is the most comfortable and useful style for women who wear a B cup or less. Bigger-bosomed women do better in encapsulator bras because they surround each mound completely and may also feature underwire for extra support. Encapsulating-type bras may seem unexciting and uninspired, but they do have one great advantage: They're far more comfortable for the bigger-breasted gal.

As with swimwear and bra styles, everyone seems to be jumping on the bandwagon to provide the best fit for our tits. Title Nine uses a nifty little barbell system to calculate the support you might need, depending on size and level of exercise. Similar companies targeting women's athletic wear, such as Athleta, also feature an easy-to-follow system to determine what bra to buy for a specific sporting activity, from low- to high-impact levels. Numerous online lingerie stores feature a wide selection of styles, sizes, and prices when it comes to sports bras. You shouldn't have to buy two inexpensive sport bras to do the job of one better-built athletic bra.

TAKE CARE OF YOUR ACTIVE WEAR

SPORTS BRAS

- Wash athletic bras in a lingerie bag, similar to a normal bra (see Chapter 2: Bras), although you may have to spend more time securing extra hooks and snaps.
- To avoid mildew, give a sweat-drenched bra room to breathe before tossing it in your laundry bag (or let it air out when you get home from the gym).
- If you participate in sports more than three or four days per week, make sure you're rotating your bras every day. The more bras you own, the longer each one will last.

SWIMWEAR

They might suffer more wear and tear than ours bras, probably because a lot of swimwear is made from more-fragile material. Ask what fabric the suit is made of before making a final purchase. Microfiber has

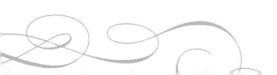

replaced cotton in most athletic wear and may be the answer to your washday prayers. Keep in mind that all the fun stuff of summer—sand, chlorine, and sun—further damage fabrics, so you'll want to take good care your suit if you plan to keep it more than one season.

- Always rinse out your suit after wearing it, especially if you've been swimming in chlorinated water.
- Never leave a wet suit wrapped up in a towel.
- Hand wash (or at the very least, put it in a lingerie bag) your suit inside out in lukewarm water.
- Always hang dry your suit out of the sun to avoid fading, and never ring out extra water by twisting and turning delicate fabric (although you can blot out excess moisture between two towels).
- Watch where you sit, since many poolside surfaces are rough and will tear fine fabrics.
- Use caution when applying body lotions and tanning sprays, since many contain chemicals that could stain your suit.
- Check the manufacturer's tags. Some brands, such as Speedo, recommend you not use any detergent, as it can break down the properties of lycra fibers.
- Consider purchasing a specially formulated swimsuit wash from a specialty swimwear store.

bOOb*flash!*

SPORTS BRA HALL OF FAME

Oprah made the ENELL Sports Bra famous by declaring it her all-time favorite. American Brandi Chastain did the same for Nike when she stripped off her jersey after making the winning play in the 1999 Women's World Soccer Cup.

EXPOSING COOPER'S DROOPERS

Many breast experts and bra manufacturers claim that wearing a sports bra while exercising will help maintain the supportive properties of our breasts' Cooper's ligaments, the dense connective tissue credited with holding it all together (fat, blood vessels, milk ducts). But when one thinks of the word "ligament," one might imagine a strong connection to a specific muscle, similar to the knee's anterior cruciate ligament. Cooper's ligaments seem to have little in common with such tough stuff, and no one seems to understand their true function. Some doctors claim they can be stretched over time, but these so-called ligaments may be no more important than our skin in keeping breasts aloft.[16] No one knows for sure what keeps our girls riding high or lying low.

IT'S GOOD FOR YOUR GIRLS, TOO

Physical exercise does benefit our breasts and has been associated with reduced rates of breast cancer in women. And participating in any type of athletic activity is good for our general health, even if we're not working out simply to lose weight. It builds flexibility, tones muscles, keeps our cardiovascular system in tip-top shape, and may slow down the body's aging clock. Dr. Roizen and Dr. Oz, authors of *You: The Owner's Manual,* calculate that a fifty-five-year-old woman who participates in regular strength and stamina activities can become 9.1 years younger than her true biological age![17] While cardio helps to keep our fat stores in balance (and thus our girls from ballooning out of proportion), toning specific muscle groups can also contribute to a perkier pair.

Many women avoid weight or strength training because they are afraid they might bulk up and look too muscular. But the opposite is true. "The average woman who lifts weights actually shrinks in body

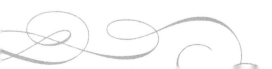

size by losing fat and shaping the muscles," says fitness expert Joan Pagano.[18] You don't have to join a gym or hire an expensive personal trainer to get started, either. Exercise balls and rubber bands that can be purchased at any drugstore are useful at-home tools to help firm and tone your body.

"Strengthening your back muscles lifts the front of your torso and opens up your chest so people can admire your beautiful bust," says fitness and wellness expert Shirley Archer. "You will look and feel more relaxed and confident, which is always sexy."[19] Her book, *Busting Out,* recommends doing simple push-up and chest press exercises two to three times per week. For a list of other fitness books and resources, see the Boobliography.

If you keep active—either by joining an athletic team, visiting your local gym, or swimming at a public pool—you'll also end up hanging around a few women's locker rooms. And that's another great side benefit to working out. You'll be exposed to the variety of sizes and shapes found among real, strong women rather than digitally created representations. This helps keep a healthy perspective on your own girls and builds an appreciation for the range and diversity of the female form.

CHAPTER SEVEN

Fully Employed Boobs: Pregnant Protrusions & Nursing Nightmares *(Or Not)*

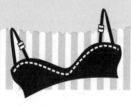

> *My boobs were huge and I was a nursing goddess. I could pump an eight-ounce bottle for my son five minutes before I walked out the door for the evening. I had no problems nursing at all.*
>
> —34C, AGE 41

> *My nipples hurt like hell. I was in such agony that I really didn't enjoy it much. Both kids ended up on formula at about two to three months because my milk supply was not adequate.*
>
> —34C, AGE 52

When we become mothers, we finally use our breasts as nature intended: to feed. During your first pregnancy, you'll probably pore over books that tout all the benefits of breastmilk, stressing that nursing provides newborns with the best start. You may be inspired by photos of calm and adorable babies suckling sweetly at their mother's breast. But like childbirth, just because something is "natural" doesn't mean you'll instinctively know how to do it without instruction. You may need to learn the rules of baby-boob engagement, so to speak. If your own experience doesn't match up to some perfect breastfeeding photo (not unlike meeting the unattainable ideal breast image), you might fear that there's something wrong with your boobs; you might feel guilty or confused. Bringing a precious new life into the world may be an immediate miracle—but adapting to baby doesn't happen overnight. Making milk and working with your baby to bring him or her this magic elixir through your breasts is also a process. If you're a new mother, give yourself time, both for your body to go through the necessary postpartum changes and to adjust to your new body afterward.

Studies show that human breastmilk is the perfect nutritional food for babies and that it helps prevent numerous diseases. We also know it's good for mom. When babies suck on the nipple *and* areola, the hormone oxytocin is released. Oxytocin works as our milk supply "let down" reflex and causes the uterus to contract and return sooner to its more pre-pregnant size.[1] Oxytocin is a feel-good hormone that assists in bonding between mother and child. Breastfeeding has also been linked to lower incidences of breast and ovarian cancers.[2] Other rewards are practical and financial in nature: It's cheaper than formula and easier to supply than mixing up a bottle in the middle of the night. Yes, it can be tiring for the new mother in the first few weeks, but its long-term benefits far outweigh short-term physical discomforts or the inconvenience of being a boob-on-call.

Worldwide health organizations, including the American Academy of Pediatrics, recommend that babies be breastfed exclusively (no

> ## MILK DOESN'T SPOUT IF AREOLA'S NOT IN MOUTH
> Time and time again, you hear lactation consultants advise nursing
> mothers to make sure the baby has a proper "latch," or hold, on the
> breast. This refers to how the baby's mouth is positioned on your
> nipple *and* areola. A correct placement assists with greater milk
> production and helps prevent sore or cracked nipples. The breast's
> milk-manufacturing system has often been described as a system of
> branches, with milk moving from the milk glands, into the ducts, and
> finally through the sinuses (where the milk pools) and out the many
> holes surrounding the nipple.[3] Compression of the sinuses is the key
> to delivering milk efficiently. In addition to the nipple, the baby's
> mouth should cover one to two inches of the areola.

solid foods or other liquids) for the first six months and that mothers continue to breastfeed for at least the first year—or until mother
and baby decide otherwise. Breastfeeding practices vary widely from
country to country, but the average global rate shows that 79 percent
of all infants are breastfed for their first twelve months of life.[4]

In the United States, breastfeeding was the norm until the twentieth century. Cow's milk was used as a substitute in the 1880s, but it
resulted in higher infant mortality rates, and mothers stopped using
it until pasteurization made milk consumption safer for babies. Over
the ensuing half century, other substitutes, including formula, were
introduced as being superior to mother's milk, and more convenient.
By 1971, breastfeeding had reached an all-time low of 24 percent. It
eventually climbed back to 51.9 percent by 1982, then dipped back
down again through the 1990s and has hovered around 70 percent
since 2002.[5] These numbers only reflect the rates at which breastfeeding is initiated. In the United States, only 33 percent of infants are
still breastfed at six months, and the number drops to 20 percent by
the time the baby is a year old.[6]

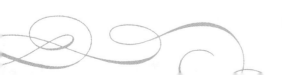

How long you decide to nurse your baby is up to you and your baby, but many physicians and health organizations encourage breast-feeding for a minimum of one year. Many mothers nurse well beyond that time, each for their own reasons. In most non-Western countries, it's not unusual to see toddlers at the breast.[7] Anthropologist Katherine Dettwyler's research shows that normal human breastfeeding can range from a low of two and a half years to a maximum of seven.[8] Human milk is perfectly suited to humans, so while there's nothing wrong with continuing to nurse for as long as it feels right for you and your child, it's important to recognize that some countries have different customs than others.

Some experts think that the low rates of breastfeeding in the United States are due to lack of education and support for breastfeeding in our society (and the way we sexualize the breast instead of honoring its true biological function). Women are often discharged from the hospital before their milk comes in and with little or no instruction or continuing follow-up on their progress. Those who return to work often find that they have no private place to pump milk during the day or that their employer doesn't allow for flexible schedules that promote continued breastfeeding. Also, as we've seen from previous chapters, our culture is divided about breastfeeding in public.

Some new moms begin with a complete commitment to breast-feeding, but stop during the first few weeks for various reasons. Some women believe this could be due, in part, to the well-intentioned public campaign to encourage women to nurse. But in the push to get new moms to stick with the program, marketing efforts can gloss over any potential problems that might occur. As one new mother explained, "I think there's a conspiracy in the medical community to keep quiet about how difficult breastfeeding can be for some women. All you hear when you're pregnant is how wonderful the experience will be, with very little information about possible problems. I had no idea how hard it was going to be." She and her spouse eventually found outside support from a lactation consultant, and she decided to supplement her nursing with formula feedings. She feels that she could have been more prepared and less surprised by her own struggle with nursing if she had been made aware of these potential complications. When a woman thinks everyone else is succeeding at breastfeeding but her, it can make her feel like a lactation failure. Disappointment in not measuring up to unreal standards causes some women to throw in the nursing towel.

BATTLE OF THE BOOBS

One of the most problematic social issues regarding breastfeeding is how often it pits one boob owner against another. Mothers who do (or did) breastfeed can make those who don't nurse for whatever reason, feel like neglectful mothers. The reasons surrounding a woman's choice to breastfeed or formula feed are often very personal. Pressure from other moms about which choice is the right choice isn't productive for women on either side of the breastfeeding divide. Maybe it's time both sides gave each other a break. Bottle-feeding moms can smile at nursing moms (instead of reporting them to management), and nursing moms can acknowledge that bottle-feeding moms are doing their best.

It can also be difficult to discuss the barriers to successful breastfeeding because everyone knows that breastmilk has huge benefits for both mother and baby, and no one wants to discourage anyone from at least trying. But each person's situation is different, and for some it's simply an impossible task. It's not always mom's fault, either. Babies can have their own problems with latching on or staying awake for long enough periods of time to stimulate breastmilk production. Monique remembers being exhausted after the birth of her two premature twins. "I used a breast pump for hours but never managed to produce more than a few drops of breastmilk." After six frustrating weeks of this routine, she finally gave up. Marisa's nipples

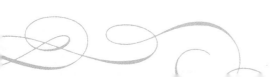

were flat and "made it impossible for my baby to latch on, resulting in forty-five-minute screaming sessions—baby screaming, me weeping." Every woman has to take into account what works—or doesn't work—for her and baby when it comes to breastfeeding.

Many women experience a profound emotional connection to their children through breastfeeding. For some, the joys of nursing are immeasurable. "Once I figured out the logistics, I was happy to let time stand still and just delight in feeding my baby," says one new mom. Another woman reflects, "Yes, I became a milk factory for my baby, but I was so in awe of my breasts. Here they were feeding my child, after having only existed prior to that for pleasing myself and my partner." One woman speaks of the physical sensation of nursing. "I can still remember the incredible physical joy, relief, release of the milk letdown—the intensity of feeling my body provide for my baby, in a manner that surpassed my mental, physical, emotional control. It's beyond comprehension to experience such a visceral response to a baby's cry."

It may be that the act of breastfeeding takes our sex back to a time when the breast was actually worshipped only for what it did best:

sustaining life outside the womb. As another mom said, "It felt so incredible that I could keep another human being alive with my own body. It made me keenly aware of the indescribable role of women in the continuance of the human race." Now, *that's* boob power.

THESE BOOBS WERE MADE FOR FEEDING

I liked having larger breasts [when I was pregnant]. I loved nursing and nursed everywhere and enjoyed the sometimes shocked looks on people's faces.
—36B, AGE 48

Mothers who breastfeed often feel self-conscious and embarrassed by the strange contradictions witnessed in a society that worships the sexualized breast but is offended by a mom who publicly nurses a hungry child. And yet no woman who discreetly (or even indiscreetly) flashes her boob in public to make an unscheduled feeding does so because she's an exhibitionist. Babies, for all their adorable qualities, determine the meal schedule.

The best way to ensure your privacy in a public place is to toss a baby blanket over your shoulder. Several manufacturers make discreet and stylish nursing tops, including bathing suits. But it's not always easy to adjust a squirmy baby into the right position, and you might find you have to expose your breast for a brief period of time until everything is in place. Some mothers have no problem with baring a breastfeeding breast. "I was—still am—pretty conservative about undressing in front of others, but when I was nursing my children, I didn't care who saw what," says one fifty-year-old mom of two. "Mine got bigger, to a C cup, and were actually a perfect size for feeding in public," says another mother.

Breastfeeding can be a source of embarrassment for other new moms. One woman recounts her experience of being in the hospital when her brother-in-law paid an unexpected visit. He sat down to chat just as her baby started fussing. She wanted to feed the baby but

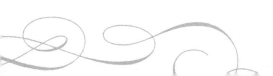

THE BABY-FRIENDLY HOSPITAL INITIATIVE

In 1991, UNICEF and the World Health Organization launched The Baby-Friendly Hospital Initiative to promote worldwide positive hospital breastfeeding practices. For a facility to be "baby-friendly," it must follow the Initiative's ten-step program,

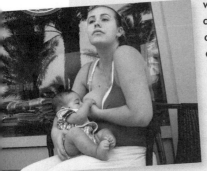

which includes educating moms about and training them to start breastfeeding; allowing baby to room-in with mom; allowing baby to breastfeed exclusively (unless otherwise medically indicated); and establishing support groups accessible to mom once she's gone home from the hospital. Since the Initiative began, more than 15,000 facilities in 134 countries have received the Baby-Friendly award.[9] In China, there are more than 6,000 Baby-Friendly Hospitals, as compared to fifty-five hospitals and birthing centers in the United States (as of September 2006).[10]

Emily Harris

realized that no man had ever seen her breasts, other than in a sexual context. Her brother-in-law kept talking as she adjusted the baby to nurse, even offering a few nursing tips from his wife's own experiences. From that moment, she says, "Breastfeeding became much more comfortable, and I was able to keep it up and really enjoy it. Who would have thought that a guy would be one of my best breastfeeding coaches?"

It could be that such a nonchalant attitude toward public nursing is exactly what's needed to help encourage women to keep breastfeeding beyond the first few months.

MAMA'S MAGICAL MILK MACHINE

Nursing was far more painful than I anticipated. I was about to give up on the idea during the second week, but that's when the pain finally started to lessen.
—36C, AGE 50

Once the baby is born, a mother's estrogen and progesterone levels drop, kicking in the milk production process. Prolactin and oxytocin step in to work their magic, the former signaling our boobs to manufacture milk and the latter working to create the let-down reflex that allows our nipples to release milk (otherwise, we'd be continuously running faucets with no shutoff valve). But breastmilk isn't present until two to five days (and sometimes longer) after birth. Instead, women's wonderful bosoms secrete a very small amount of a substance called colostrum, which some people refer to as pre-milk. It's thought to have special properties that help ready an infant's intestines for the milk that soon will be available.[11]

Mothers should be encouraged to have skin-to-skin contact with their baby as soon as possible after birth and to begin nursing within an hour or two of birth so that the newborn will benefit from the vitamin-rich colostrum. Over the following few days, as the milk "comes in," a new mother's breasts will become even larger and firmer than before. Sometimes there is too much milk production and breasts become "engorged," which can result in pain and difficulty with nursing. Women should get instruction in how to nurse their newborn before leaving the hospital. Even then, many women find that they need additional professional support once they're home and the real milk-making begins.

Milk production is ruled by the law of supply and demand. The more your baby sucks at the breast, the more milk you produce. And since newborn babes have very small stomachs, they may want to nurse as often as every one to three hours. The American Academy

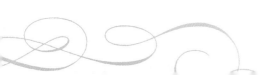

of Pediatrics advises new mothers to nurse eight to twelve times in a twenty-four-hour period. They also advise that no pacifiers or other substitutes, such as water or formula, be introduced. This is recommended to avoid "nipple confusion," so that the baby's sucking reflex is solely focused on pumping mom's milk supply. But every baby is different. Some can use a pacifier all day and still nurse efficiently at their mother's breast. Others can't handle anything but the real thing. You'll have to watch your own infant closely and determine what works best for the two of you. You want to ensure that your baby's getting enough time at your breast to get the milk production running smoothly and efficiently.

Some babies can become breastfeeding experts in just a few days, while others may take as long as two to six weeks to master the breast. Different positions may help make things easier, so it's worthwhile to learn about other ways to present your boob to your new baby, including while you're lying down.[12] Some new moms have problems with cracked or sore nipples. Experts advise alleviating such pain by correcting the latch the baby has on the breast. In other cases, physical problems, such as blocked ducts, can complicate the entire process. Once breastfeeding is firmly established, you'll nurse fewer times per day. It should take approximately ten minutes for your baby to empty each breast. (This is also about the same amount of time it takes for an effective electric breast pump to empty your breasts.) But remember, just like our boobs, no two babies are alike. As your own unique infant grows and changes, you might breastfeed more or less often than another mom. You may think you aren't producing enough milk, but it could be that your baby is nursing more often because she's experiencing a sudden growth spurt. Pediatricians agree that steady weight gain is the best measure of nursing success.

SUCKLING SUPPORT

*My breasts were so heavy that I had to nurse lying down,
and my areola would smother my daughter so I had
to make sure she could always breathe!*
—44DD, AGE 35

Many moms start out with the breast of intentions when it comes to nursing their babies but can often become overwhelmed if any problems arise. It's best to prepare ahead of time if you're planning on sticking to a breastfeeding regimen. Keep breastfeeding support hotlines handy, or read up on websites such as La Leche League, which assist breastfeeding mothers. Many new mothers get support from breastfeeding blogs written by other new moms. Your obstetrician or pediatrician can also refer you to a local breastfeeding support group, and most hospitals have outpatient clinics where you can bring your baby for a visit should you have questions or problems. You might also consider hiring a private lactation consultant who can come to your home, although hourly rates start at $150 and up, so it's certainly not an affordable option for everyone. Some of these charges may (and should) be reimbursed by insurance.

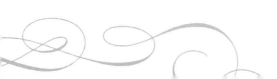

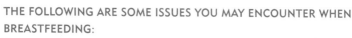

THE FOLLOWING ARE SOME ISSUES YOU MAY ENCOUNTER WHEN
BREASTFEEDING:

Engorgement

Some women find their breasts so full that it's impossible to nurse. Cold packs and massage often help alleviate this situation. Pumping can help, too, but it can also cause more problems by increasing milk supply. Engorgement can also be relieved by switching nursing positions.

Inverted, Flat, or Novice Nipples

There's no good way to "toughen up" nipples, and some women have more-sensitive skin than others. Bleeding and cracked nipples hurt, which also makes nursing more difficult. The first remedy is to try to correct the baby's latch. For relief, pure lanolin may help (although not if you are allergic to wool), as can hydrogel pads. For inverted or flat nipples, you can try silicone nipple shields or breast shells that help push the nipple outward. Though nipple shields were once controversial, studies now show that they don't reduce a woman's milk supply and that they can be very helpful for moms with premature babies who have developmental issues associated with sucking.[13]

Slow, Sleepy, or Fussy Eaters

Babies come in all temperaments. Many moms have to wake up sleepy babies to ensure that they are eating at least every four hours during the first few days and weeks. Other babies might be fussy or prefer one breast to the other. Many new moms complain that their breasts become lopsided because baby likes one side best.

Breast Infections: Plugged Milk Ducts, Mastitis, Breast Abscesses, and Lumps

Some women experience occasional plugged milk ducts, which may be relieved by warm compresses and massage. Around 30 percent of nursing mothers may end up with mastitis, which is a bacterial infection that can be treated with antibiotics. Moms will usually run a fever and have flu-like symptoms. On occasion, a breast infection can lead to a breast abscess, which must be drained by a surgeon. Other oddities include lumpy breasts, which can be normal but should still be checked by a physician.[14] None of these conditions should prevent a woman from nursing, but they can make it more uncomfortable.

bOOb*flash!*

BIGGER BREASTS DON'T PRODUCE LARGER QUANTITIES OF MILK

They simply contain more fat. All breasts—regardless of size—contain the equipment needed to function as self-contained milk machines, which include fifteen to twenty-five different milk lobes inside each breast. Petite girls may find their size is an advantage in nursing. Experts believe that a small- to medium-size-boob owner may have an easier time positioning her baby and getting a good latch.

OTHER ASSORTED ISSUES

Women who have had breast reduction surgery or other surgical procedures may face some challenges with breastfeeding, many of which can be resolved with proper assistance. Mothers of twins or premature babies, or those facing additional medical obstacles, may find it useful to contact a professional or other support organization. Women who sport nipple rings should remove them before nursing, and some report that these extra holes can cause added leaking.

Relying on several nursing resources (whether it's books, websites, support groups, professionals, or just positive and encouraging

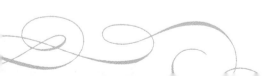

SAGGY-BOOB EFFECTS

Does breastfeeding cause breasts to sag? That may be a matter of perception. An Italian study found that 73 percent of mothers thought their breasts had changed due to pregnancy, either because they got bigger or lost firmness. All participants thought their boobs had changed in one way or another, even if they hadn't breastfed.[15]

Just getting pregnant makes a difference to our breasts—whether or not we end up nursing a child. If you experience greater weight gain and loss during pregnancy, you will also experience more loose skin around your breasts. Every woman carries her weight differently and has individual skin elasticity to contend with. Many women report that their breasts lose volume once they stop nursing but that some of the bounce returns to their boobs after a few more months have passed. Other women prefer their post-nursing breasts. Most simply get used to the new way their boobs look and are fine with their differently shaped breasts. Some who are very unhappy with how their breasts look after pregnancy and/or nursing might opt for plastic surgery (see Chapter 11: Cut and Paste).

friends) can make many of the above problems seem like small bumps along the breastfeeding road. Even with all this help, though, there may be situations in which nursing exclusively is just not possible. According to Dr. Susan Love, "Sometimes a combination of breastfeeding and bottle-feeding (using either formula or breastmilk expressed by the mother at an earlier time) can be a useful compromise."[16]

MAMMARY MILK MYTHS

Nursing prevents pregnancy. Don't count on it. While studies show that if you follow some very strict breastfeeding guidelines (including nursing around-the-clock exclusively, with no pacifiers or bottles), this method is still not 100 percent effective.[17] Just because you're not having periods doesn't mean you can't get pregnant while nursing.

Babies who breastfeed have higher IQs. This is often quoted as a statement of fact, but recent research shows that a mother's own IQ has more to do with her baby's intelligence than the quality of her breastmilk.[18]

Women who can't nurse just aren't trying hard enough. While making an extra effort can often be the key to breastfeeding success, there are some cases in which it's simply not possible. Some moms have insufficient lactation tissue (as in the case of tubular breasts), or a baby might be born with some other physical disability that interferes with her ability to breastfeed. While these are rare cases, it's still important to remember to be flexible and seek help early on if you feel you are having any difficulties.

UNBELIEVABLE BOOBS

It was during my three pregnancies that I finally got boobs! It was only with age and added weight that I've maintained them.

−36C, age 52

"My breasts let me know I was pregnant—they were so sore," says one thirty-year-old 36D. When the hormones estrogen and progesterone increase, tissue begins to swell, and your boobs may be painful. Sometimes it hurts to roll onto them in bed, and you might not be so thrilled by the idea of anyone touching that part of your anatomy. During pregnancy, a woman's boobs grow quickly and are often hard, and the nipples darken, and become more prominent, while the areola becomes larger.[19] Some women develop stretch marks from rapidly expanding skin. Nipples can become supersensitive, which can be either a good or bad thing, depending on the individual.

Not everyone reacts to this boob enhancement in the same way. "My breasts grew to a 36EE, but my belly was so big that for the first time my breasts looked smaller," says a petite 34D. One woman, who felt her breasts had been "gnat bites" before pregnancy, was thrilled at their new size. "My breasts became huge, a 38C, and I loved them. I

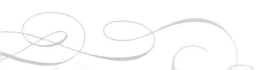

had cleavage for the first time in my life." One 34B woman who wasn't accustomed to wearing bras had mixed feelings. "When I got pregnant, my breasts got huge and I had to wear a bra. I admit I sort of enjoyed having big ones for a while. I got to see what it was like to have men stare at my boobs. But I soon grew tired of that and was happy to go back to my braless ways." No two women will have the same experience with their breasts. And with each succeeding pregnancy, they may get larger or smaller and change size and shape again.

PUT YOUR BEST BREAST FORWARD

Mine didn't change much, but I loved feeling like there was a purpose for these things I had been hauling around for years. Until my daughter was born, my breasts—and butt—were out of proportion to my waist; I had to tailor all my slacks and skirts. Afterward, my stomach wasn't as flat and clothes fit better.

—36F, AGE 46

Breastfeeding is often called an "art." But even the most talented artist isn't always recognized for the physical effort involved in creating a particular masterpiece. Many artistic endeavors are only realized after a lot of hard work. As a new mom, you are in a similar position, except you're physically and mentally exhausted from having just given birth. Then there's this wonderful creature who's suddenly completely dependent on you. Even if you've read numerous (and often contradictory) instruction books, it's often tough to figure out who's in charge once you're home with your new baby. Breastfeeding isn't the only new learning activity you might be focused on. In addition to diapers, bathing, and dressing, there's all that baby equipment, too. Just figuring out whether the car seat is in the right position is enough to give some new parents nightmares. And, of course, you're functioning on three to four hours of sleep per night. Breastfeeding can be an enjoyable and very fulfilling part of motherhood, if you—and your partner—are prepared and know what to anticipate.

BEST BRAS FOR YOUR BODACIOUS BREASTS

Your breasts can double or triple in size when you're pregnant. In addition, your rib cage expands to make room for your growing baby. Good maternity and nursing bras are made to hold your heavier breasts, and are equipped with extra rows of hooks. Nursing bras were once thought to interfere with milk production and possibly cause blocked ducts, but today's flexible underwire maternity bras offer the best support. Toward the end of your pregnancy, around your eighth month, you'll want to invest in three good nursing bras. At a minimum, you want one to wear and one to spare, while the third will typically be in the wash. Some women also choose to wear a cotton nursing bra at night.

Pick a design that allows you to easily and quickly expose a breast with only one hand. (Remember, you'll be holding a hungry baby!) Manufacturers now offer more styles and selections in larger sizes, so check out online maternity and nursing websites for the best selection (see the Boobliography). Bella Materna makes beautiful maternity and nursing bras in sizes 32C to 49G. Owner Anne Diamond believes that nursing moms who feel pretty in their foundations are more likely to enjoy the experience and possibly breastfeed longer. "Enough is changing in a new mom's world," says Anne. "She should be able to choose bras that are functional but still retain her personal style."[20]

There seems to be a trend toward offering more-enticing maternity and nursing wear for women, which may be due to the latest celebrity baby boom. Singer Gwen Stefani wore fashion-forward nursing bras from lingerie maker Agent Provocateur after the birth of her son. Whatever you choose to wear, don't forget to buy disposable or reusable cloth nursing pads to protect your fabulous new lingerie wardrobe!

How do you spell breastfeeding success? S-U-P-P-O-R-T.

Start early. Sign up for pre-natal breastfeeding classes, or contact your local La Leche League for groups in your area. Inquire about your hospital's breastfeeding policies and determine if they are "Baby-Friendly" (see sidebar earlier in this chapter). Talk to your obstetrician and ask for any breastfeeding resources or referrals. Visit friends and family who are breastfeeding, or who have breastfed, and talk to them about their experiences.

Understand that breastfeeding is a learning process for you and your baby. It can be very frustrating if your baby doesn't take to your breast easily. Make sure you have the name and number of a good lactation professional or other helpful on-call service to whom you can ask questions. Remember, some babies can have developmental issues that interfere with the nursing process.

Prepare your home or workplace. Make sure you have a cozy and comfortable place to nurse your baby. Consider purchasing a nursing pillow, or a stool for your feet. Stock up on supplies, including those for sore nipples, and nursing pads to catch spilled milk. If you must return to work right away, figure out what the workplace breastfeeding policies are and plan a quiet and discreet pumping station. Consider renting an electric pump while you are still at home, both to adjust to the new routine and to ensure a faster and more effective way to express your milk. Stock up on all the necessary supplies to keep and store your breastmilk.

Practice patience. Every boob and baby bond uniquely. If you become anxious about your breastfeeding experience, take a break and contact a specialist, or talk with other nursing moms. You don't need to follow anyone else's nursing agenda but your own.

Overcome perfection. You may have to supplement with formula on occasion or introduce a pacifier to meet your baby's intense sucking needs. Remember that the longer you continue to nurse, the better it is for you and baby. Don't give up completely just because you can't breastfeed at every feeding. Set realistic goals that make sense for you.

Remember to ask for help. You may be the sole milk provider, but that doesn't mean your partner or spouse can't play a valuable and supportive role. Your partner can help out by making sure you're well hydrated and comfortable and by observing and/or helping baby get into a proper nursing position. He or she can also attend breastfeeding classes or observe videos and websites about proper breastfeeding practice and potential problems.

Take care of yourself. Your body is working around the clock. You'll need to eat right and drink plenty of water. Accept offers from friends and family in the first few weeks, whether it's to provide the occasional nutritious meal or to give you a break while you take a long shower or a much-needed nap. Purchase a small battery-operated pump for occasional expression of milk so you know you can take a short nursing break once in a while.

CHAPTER EIGHT

Lovers Love 'Em: Sharing Your Breast Self

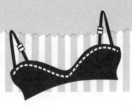

My sister and I both concur that many boys/men out there don't know how much we women just enjoy a little boob time once in a while. My lover gladly bestows attention on my breasts, and he has always said he loves them, which makes me feel more like a woman for the appreciation I receive toward my body.
—36C, AGE 21

I like the way they look, and I get a lot of positive feedback from my partner about them. They're a huge part of my sexual satisfaction.
—38C, AGE 33

Advertisers know that they stir sexual appetites when they place female breasts in their campaigns. It's a come-on, a tease, a way to get our attention. And it works. But, as highlighted in previous chapters, the focus on perfect, young breasts can also have the effect of making some women uncomfortable with their own bodies. Remember, those idealized images do not resemble society's norm, and comparing our breasts to those plastered on billboards or in magazines does nothing to help our own self-image. It's ironic in a way, because breast admirers know that the soft, natural curves of women's bosoms are alluring and seductive specifically because they're both sexual and nurturing. In the context of a loving, fulfilling sexual relationship, breasts should bring joy to boob owners and partners alike. And when women feel proud of their own breasts, they are more comfortable sharing the pleasures their breasts have to offer.

SEX AND THE BREAST:
LEARNED OR INTUITIVE BEHAVIOR

I love them! My best friend is also my life partner, and I love to look at her breasts and relax into their wonderful softness.
−38C, AGE 33

My boyfriend loves to lie on me. He says my chest makes for a great pillow, and he can hear my heartbeat through them, which makes him feel super comfortable.
−52GG, AGE 20

Straight, gay, bi, transgender—no matter your inclination, everyone recognizes that breasts are a symbol of sexuality in Western societies. There are cultures that don't sexualize breasts, but that's certainly not the case in the United States. And while breasts have been romanticized and adored for centuries as part of the beauty of a woman, they did not reach their more sexually charged iconic status until the twentieth century. Maybe it's due to our history of legislatively curtailing the sight of our Nipples of Mass Distraction, or perhaps it's the way we've marketed the breast to become singularly sexual. There's no room for breastfeeding in public when nudity is categorized as "adult entertainment." The message is clear: Naked breasts induce (unsolicited) sexual arousal.

It could be that we only derive sexual pleasure from breasts, whether as owners or onlookers, because our society views them as sexual. Anthropologist Katherine Dettwyler spent years researching breastfeeding practices in other cultures and believes this is the case. According to her, "Physiological responses such as sexual arousal are conditioned by social assumptions."[1] In societies like Mali, where breasts are openly displayed and nursing is viewed as ordinary, such nudity isn't associated with sexual arousal. Interestingly, there isn't much in the way of statistical evidence regarding women's preferences for breast play. While many women consider their breasts an important erogenous zone, others do not. It could be that it only feels good to have our breasts caressed because we've been told we should enjoy it.

Alfred Kinsey, founder of the scientific study of human sexuality, first published *Sexual Behavior in the Human Female* in 1953, the first examination of its kind. Kinsey and his staff conducted interviews with more than eighteen thousand men and women and found that half of all females viewed their breasts as erotically sensitive. In less than 1 percent of the women surveyed, breast stimulation alone was enough to experience the Big O. (Wouldn't life be grand if it were that easy for the rest of us?) Kinsey also found that the fondling of breasts ranked second only to kissing as the most important aspect of foreplay.[2] More than fifty years have passed since Kinsey's report, and today many more women believe their breasts are an important part of sex. In a 2006 study, 82 percent of young women believed their sexual arousal was caused or enhanced by breast stimulation, while 7.5 percent thought it decreased their sexual pleasure. If

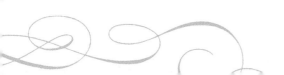

touching a woman's breasts, or having them touched, is a culturally learned response, why are some men aroused by having *their* nipples fondled? In the same study, 52 percent of men enjoyed having their nipples stimulated, while about 8 percent considered it a turn-off.[5]

The answer to this nip conundrum could rest in our bodies' ability to produce a nifty little hormone named oxytocin (not to be confused with the narcotic oxycodone, or OxyContin, made famous by nationally known broadcasting boob).[6] Oxytocin is best known for inducing labor by stimulating uterine contractions. But it also stimulates the ejection of a mother's breastmilk after she's given birth and is released in the body of males and females during orgasm. It's been called the "love" or "bonding" hormone, because it's thought to facilitate emotional bonding between mother and child. Its presence during sex also supports that idea since it suggests that it's an important part of bonding with a lover.[7] Levels of oxytocin, which can be measured in the blood, rise when a woman's nipples are stimulated, even if she isn't pregnant or lactating.[8] It's unclear whether men experience the same hormonal release when their nipples are rubbed the right way, since no studies could be found that measure their levels of the hormone during such activity.

Sexual arousal may also be related to our breasts' blood supply and sensitive connective tissue. Dr. Miriam Stoppard, author of *101 Essential Tips: Breast Care,* writes that women's breasts are classified as one of our primary erogenous zones, together with lips, buttocks, and our

bOOb*flash!*

PREGNANT NIPPLE ALERT

Physicians sometimes warn that stimulating the nipples of a pregnant woman can induce uterine contractions, which could theoretically cause the early onset of labor. Though oxytocin is used in its synthetic form to jumpstart labor, or continue a lapsed labor, it has not been proven that stimulating women's breasts produces enough of the hormone to actually begin or keep labor going for any length of time.[9]

external genital organs. Since our breasts contain numerous nerves, they can be responsive to touch, pain, and temperature.[10] Breasts can enlarge as much as 25 percent during sex. This enlargement is temporary and is not seen in women who have breastfed, although the reason isn't clear[11]—yet another of the many mysteries about women's breasts. In many women, a rush of blood to the breasts during sex results in the skin reacting as it would to exercise or vigorous activity, resulting in what is known as a "sexual flush."[12]

Given that breasts are as sexualized as they are in our culture, along with the fact that many women find breasts an important part of their sexuality, you would think that popular how-to sex books would devote a great deal of print to their stimulation. Quite the contrary. In the four-hundred-plus-page *Sex for Dummies,* by Dr. Ruth Westheimer, one of the most noted sexperts in the business, only a few sentences are devoted to breasts as a source of sexual arousal. More attention is paid to breast cancer, breastfeeding, and the evils of breast enhancement than to the physical pleasure that may be given or received from

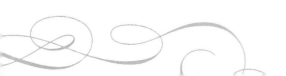

a woman's breast.[13] *Sex: A Man's Guide,* brought to us by the editors of *Men's Health* magazine, doesn't have much to say about stimulation and arousal, either. In the mere 5 pages, out of 656, devoted to breasts, the authors advise: "Don't kneed them like bread. Adore them."[14] The *Guide to Getting It On,* by Paul Joannides and Daerick Gross, does a little bit better, featuring illustrations and detailed instruction and devoting an entire chapter to nipples alone. It includes such wise advice as paying attention to both breasts and informs readers that there are no hard and fast rules when it comes to nipple sensitivity and breast size. They suggest adapting your style of breast play from boob owner to boob owner. They recognize that every woman enjoys a different type of breast stimulation, depending on her unique pair. But don't think that it's all about the nipple. (Even though urbandictionary.com lists "Tune in Tokyo" as a game of nipple stimulation, it's also defined as excessive—and potentially painful—breast play.) Breast tissue reaches from the clavicle bone, down to our ribs, and then over and under our armpits. Lots of women would be extremely pleased if more attention were paid to that entire territory.

For some women, breast play is all the rage, while others have little sensitivity in that region and don't get what the big deal is all about. But any woman's breasts, especially unclothed, are a beautiful sight to behold. They are soft, warm, inviting pillows of flesh. For our lovers, that alone should make them irresistible.

PASTIES AND OTHER PECULIAR PECCADILLOES

Pasties or tassels: Burlesque is back, both onstage and in the bedroom. Nip coverings can be made from all types of materials: plastic, feathers, and even crystals. If you only think of pasties as evocative of sexual play, you'll miss their ability to keep you legally covered. The inexpensive stick-on variety are easy to attach or remove, and can be worn in the water (although they won't stick to oiled or sunscreened breasts). More-traditional pasties, often in heavier fabric or featuring tassels, require the use of spirit gum or some other liquid adhesive to keep them in place. Make sure to build in some clean-up time to remove any trace of less-than-appetizing bonding agents from your breasts.

Molly Crabapple

Nipple jewelry: Nipple piercing has been popular with both men and women for centuries. Nipple jewelry, to adorn and enhance the beauty of the breast, includes chains, rings, and shields. Chains can be worn between two already ring-pierced nipples, or you can choose from nonpiercing varieties that simply attach to the nipple by fitting snugly around them. Rings and shields go through an opening at the nipples' base, and their prime purpose is to keep a woman's nipples constantly erect. Shields usually cover more of the areola, with the nipple protruding from a hole in the middle. Rings come in all shapes and can dangle down like earrings. The nipple shield achieved instant infamy at the 2004 Super Bowl, when it was exposed during Janet Jackson's wardrobe malfunction.

SuzyLamont.com

Nipple clamps: Nipple clamps are used to pinch the nipples in order to obtain a degree of sexual arousal. Some are linked by a chain; others have metal or rubber tip coverings. You can even purchase multispeed vibrating nipple clamps! Some also have a mechanism to adjust the pressure and tightness. It is advised that clamps be used for short periods of time (somewhere between five and ten minutes), since they can reduce circulation.

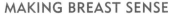

MAKING BREAST SENSE

My breasts aren't very sensitive, so I tend to ignore them.
I'd rather men focus on other areas of my body.
—36C, AGE 22

I'm large breasted, and I've always loved it when my partner makes
love to my tits. I actually get a lot of sensation along my sternum, so
when there's a lot of moving back and forth there, it feels great.
—34DDD, AGE 42

Though many women don't care to be defined by their breasts, plenty of us embrace our girls as an important part of erotic pleasure. But, again, degree and intensity vary depending on the individual boob owner. There's no rhyme or reason as to why some women have greater, lesser, or zero sensitivity in their breasts or nipples. Shape and size don't seem to matter. Even if touching feels good to our breasts during sexual foreplay, it may reach a point of overstimulation and lose its appeal. For other women, fondling their own breasts is an essential component of masturbation. Some women also enjoy accessories to supplement their sexual experience—like nipple clamps. But there will always be a segment of the female population that doesn't

---

BREAST PLEASURE OR PAIN?

How a woman reacts to breast play depends on the individual and her breasts. Any of the following could be viewed as welcome or annoying, depending on the boob owner: biting, blowing, caressing, flicking, fondling, grabbing, kissing, licking, massaging, oiling, pinching, rubbing, slapping, stroking, sucking, squeezing, touching, thrusting, tracing, or tweaking. Be sure to tell your partner what you do and don't enjoy.

get off on any of the above and wish their partners would focus on other erogenous zones to peak their libidos. Whatever your personal preferences, do what's right for you. When it comes to individual boob proclivities, you make the rules.

Breast sensations change during the course of a woman's lifetime. A shy young girl may have a perkier set of breasts but be more sexually inhibited and unable to realize their pleasures. Another woman with less bounce but more years to her bust may be confidently aware of her breast needs. Some women find the fullness experienced in pregnancy as sensual and nurturing, while others temporarily lose interest in any type of breast play. Many women experience heightened or lessened nipple sensation during and after breastfeeding. Breast surgeries can also impact sensitivity, either increasing such responses or eliminating them altogether.

A woman's sensitivity isn't dependant solely on surface arousal. Negative statements about breasts can impact our self-esteem and impact our experience. Positive statements have the effect of making us feel valued not just for our breasts, but their unique qualities. Maddie smiles as she relates how her husband "tells me his favorite part of my breast is the soft underside." Another woman recalls a girlfriend she once had who curled up beside her and laid her head on her DD breasts. She would tell her, "This is my happy place." Kathy's first boyfriend used to talk to her breasts. "He didn't name them or anything, but he would whisper things to them and tell me what they wanted, which was generally to be 'free, free, FREE!' I know it sounds lame, but it was incredibly cute at the same time. He would just hold them sometimes, which was surprisingly comforting." While most of these mammoirs have little to do with sex or foreplay, they speak volumes to how the sexual breast can be nurturing, comforting, and sensual—all in one attractive package. It's important to tell a woman how much joy her breasts provide, especially (or even) when they're fully dressed.

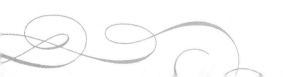

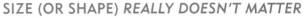

SIZE (OR SHAPE) *REALLY DOESN'T MATTER*

*In my experience, guys are so happy to be in the presence of naked
boobs that they don't notice how big, small, or lopsided they are.*

—36C, AGE 36

Since busty women seem to be the focus of advertisers, they can also
receive a larger—and often unwanted—share of male attention for
their attributes. But many small-breasted women understand that the
media preference for bigger boobs has nothing to do with the reality
of sexual attraction. "The greatest thing I ever heard about my A cup
boobs was from my husband while we were dating," Michelle recalls.
"He told me, 'Well, you might not have the biggest boobs in the
world, but you definitely have the nicest tits I've ever seen!'"

Most smaller-busted women speak to the idea that whatever less-
than-perfect thoughts we might have about our own size and shape
don't seem to matter to our partners. "He loves my breasts and says
they're the best he's ever seen," relates Amy, a fifty-one-year-old A
cup. One self-conscious young lady was put at ease by a man who
told her that her boobs were "just perfect" after she apologized for
how saggy she thought they were. It's freeing to be able to set aside
our insecurities when we're in the company of someone who enjoys
us, especially if that feeling is reciprocal. "The most wonderful thing
a partner can do is not make me feel self-conscious about them," says
Susan, a twenty-eight-year-old A cup. "If someone enjoys them, I feel
better about them and don't care that I'm not more voluptuous."

Since our breasts are always changing, it's nice to know that
they're accepted, and even appreciated, for their innately unpredict-
able natures. Bob says, "I have only had one lover, my now-wife, who
was my girlfriend when we met at fifteen. I have always loved her
breasts: small, and now larger, after all these years." Even women who
surgically alter their breasts confirm that such changes have more to

do with how they feel about their own breasts than how others feel about them. "My husband was just as happy with my saggy boobs before I had my breast lift," points out Patricia. Andrea didn't get her breasts until the age of forty, when she underwent sex-change surgery. She says, "My husband always tells me how beautiful my breasts are."

While minor physical flaws can be bothersome or make us self-conscious, these concerns pale in comparison to how our breast land-scape might appear after treatment for breast cancer. For some, this means the loss of one or both breasts, scarred and rebuilt breasts, or a lumpectomy resulting in two different sizes or shapes of breasts. Some women seem to find the silver linings to these situations, too. Amy remembers, "The first man I showed my lumpectomy scar to was my best male friend. He asked me if he could see it and gently ran his hands along the shallow, straight scar. He reassured me that it was beautiful, that I was beautiful, and that the cancer souvenir wouldn't matter to the right person. I've remained grateful for his wise words and repeat them out loud to myself whenever doubt creeps in—usually on the brink of an encounter with a new prospect. But, I look at my body in the mirror and cup my gorgeous breast, knowing I've got a built-in way to Weedwack all the Mr. Wrongs out of my life."

Reconstructing Aphrodite, a photographic compilation of twenty-seven top-free breast cancer survivors who had breast reconstructions, is a graphic example of how breast nudity can take on an entirely new meaning.[15] In nearly every photo you can feel the strength these survivors convey, not because of their rebuilt breasts, but because of what radiates from the page: confident women who are willing to share the beauty of their breasts, even if scarred. Many of these women relate how their closest and most intimate relationships helped get them through difficult times. One thirty-five-year-old model shares, "My husband was a big support—he made it a lot easier for me. We knew we were going to stay married—with a breast, without a breast—it didn't matter."[16]

Not all women choose breast reconstruction, and the absence of flesh on their torsos does not take away from their femininity or sexuality. We are who we are underneath it all, and our breasts are merely symbols of the inner qualities we possess. While we may admire or even envy the beauty of some breasts, we recognize that a woman's worth is greater than the sum of her body parts.

BELOVED BOSOMS

The discovery of breasts is the fun part. Every woman's breasts are as different as her likes, dislikes, and preferences—and that is the joy of courting.

—MALE, AGE 31

Ironically, many people think lesbians choose to be with women because they have some penis phobia. For me, I'm with a woman because I appreciate that she has what a man doesn't . . . breasts! I also take pleasure in knowing that my breasts bring pleasure to her.

—38C, AGE 46

Women may be the last to comprehend the true beauty that others see reflected on our chests. One thirty-one-year-old male doesn't get women's negative dialogue about their own breasts. "Women with small breasts seem to self-deprecate more, and this frustrates me. It's hard to hear that kind of talk from a woman you think is incredibly beautiful and sexy." Unfortunately, we may not believe those who bestow such praise, thinking that they are blinded by love and/or lust. We might not be able to treasure even the most sincere compliment.

Sometimes we need to take a look at our own breasts from a different perspective. Jackie, age fifty, says, "As a lesbian, I love nice breasts. My partner has a great rack, which I completely appreciate!

It was in coming to awareness and embracing my sexual orientation, in my forties, that I came to more fully appreciate my own breasts. Breasts are an important aspect of lesbian intimacy—and play a central role in intimate, sexual exchange." When we see the beauty in another woman's breast, we learn to love our own even more.

A gentle first encounter goes a long way toward helping us accept ourselves, too. Christine, a twenty-six-year-old B cup, had heard tales of crass guys with less-than-gentle fondling techniques, absent of any emotion or real intimacy. "The first time I had a guy caress my boob on a date, I was startled," she says, "but he was very tender and it was a good experience." So while negative comments from intimate partners can sting and damage our breast self-esteem, meeting up with someone who does appreciate our boob qualities changes the equation. Lilly, age eighteen, recalls, "After being told my nipples were too large, the best thing that anyone ever said about my breasts was that they loved my nipples." Sometimes we're able to move forward on our own and come to terms with the breast flaws we, or some inconsiderate individual, perceive.

It can be difficult for women to believe that men aren't more sexually attracted to the porn star look that's available at the click of a mouse. True, bigger boobs are attention grabbing, but there's a big difference between fantasy and reality. Some people are fascinated by big boobs, but that doesn't mean that everyone who looks at big boobs necessarily expects that in their partners. On the other hand, porn can play into some people's desires in a negative way. A study of university students showed that prolonged consumption of pornography led to greater dissatisfaction with an intimate partner's appearance.[17] If your guy or gal appears addicted to porn or Internet sex, be warned that his or her view of your body (and breasts) may become distorted. Women who indulge in such fantasies can also skew their physical perceptions of men, since these findings pertained to both sexes.

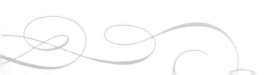

IT'S A BOOBIESEXUAL WORLD

The term "boobiesexual" was coined by the podcaster Cunning Minx and refers to "women who are mostly straight but who are really, really into women's breasts." Columnist Rachel Kramer Bussel expanded the definition to include gay men, because, although they're committed to their own sexual orientation, many are still really turned on by the sight of women's breasts.[18] As one gay man states, "Have you ever seen a drag queen with small tits? All men love breasts." Boobiesexual men and women are aroused by breasts but don't necessarily want to have sex with the women who wear them. Here's one more category of breast admiration in a world where every inclination is branded with a unique label.

No matter their size or shape dressing our girls up just to take them out can be a real turn-on. Whether your tastes run in the direction of lace or leather, there's nothing more enticing than wearing a garment that begs to be removed (for all the right reasons, of course). Rebecca Apsan, owner of La Petite Coquette in New York and author of *The Lingerie Handbook,* calls it "dressing to undress." She says that even women who don't feel like they have the body to wear lingerie should do so for that very reason. "It lets you highlight what you want to display and hide what you want to downplay," says Apsan.[19] Some women might want to try donning either a corset or a bustier. They can smooth out body flaws and accentuate and uplift their positives. As an added bonus, studies show that 75 percent of all men like lacy lingerie.[20] Sexy bras, camisoles, and negligees can make some women feel more attractive and feminine. And if it puts you in an amorous mood, how can that *not* inspire a lover?

Picking out something that you and your partner both love may be easier than you think. Men especially can be baffled by all the options available. Luckily, we live in an era when just about every

BREAST PLATTERS: WHO DOES THE DISHES?

Sex and food have much in common. Both satisfy bodily urges and meet our need for immediate gratification. And sharing a meal with someone can create a sense of intimacy and bonding (not to mention that many edibles, like oysters, are also considered aphrodisiacs). Just think of all the words for food that are used to describe breasts. (See the sidebar Tasty T(r)eats in Chapter 1.) It may speak to women's unique ability to feed our young, or maybe it just implies that our girls are good enough to eat.

And what to make of breasts as literal service platters? Maybe we should blame the Baby Boomer generation, which could have been unduly influenced by the 1965 album cover *Whipped Cream and Other Delights*, by Herb Alpert & Tijuana Brass, which features a young woman's breasts (and body) covered in—you guessed it—whipped cream. Or it might have been the 1986 food-as-foreplay film *9 1/2 Weeks*, starring Mickey Rourke and Kim Basinger. In 2004, Chinese authorities stopped a Beijing restaurant from serving sushi on women's naked bodies.[21]

Whatever the origin, some lovers enjoy covering women's breasts with a variety of toppings: from fluffy confections to chocolate sauce, honey, yogurt, and other sweet delights. Not everyone enjoys the mess that comes with these culinary entertainments, but plenty find the eroticism and fun are worth it. Angela recalls a boyfriend who "made sure that whenever we had ice cream at home, the girls got some, too. He would also lovingly clean them. I'm not really sure whose benefit this was for, but I felt it was a nice policy of breast inclusion."

mall in American invites both men and women to look at and touch the latest in adventurous underthings. Victoria's Secret offers both everyday and flirty boudoir selections in bras, panties, and sleepwear. Make a date with your partner and show him or her exactly what you find attractive and sexually appealing. Walk around the store together and see what catches your mutual attention. For some inspiration, fill out "A Lover's Guide to My Girls," below. You'll want to make sure your partner knows what colors and styles flatter your figure most. Smaller lingerie boutiques often offer enough privacy that you can try on and model selections for your paramour. Check your local boutique lingerie listings for the store nearest you.

Even if you fit within the limited sizes offered in department or specialty stores, you may want to surf the web for items that are more unique or exotic. If you go online, invite your sweetie to join you for a cyber excursion into the wild world of lingerie. Just about anything is imaginable when you have the whole world at your fingertips. You can bookmark your favorite sites and fill in size and shipping choices. (Tip: Surprise your partner by paying extra and choosing the quickest method of delivery.) For a list of web lingerie retailers and manufacturers, see the Boobliography.

A LOVER'S GUIDE TO MY GIRLS

Need a way to express your breast preferences? Fill out the following questions and consider sharing it with your favorite intimate.

- Bra size: _____
- Favorite bra color and material: _____
- What I like to hear about them: _____
- What you should never say about them: _____
- Breast activities I enjoy: _____
- Combo moves that work for me: _____
- Things I'd like to try: _____
- What I like best about my breasts: _____

_____
_____
_____

NOTE: THIS IS ALSO AVAILABLE FOR DOWNLOAD AT WWW.BOOKSONBOOBS.COM.

CHAPTER NINE

Your Breast Potential: The Path to Better Boob Well-Being

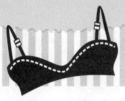

[During] my first mammogram I was scared to death. I have three older sisters who basically told me, "It sucks"—that's how they explained periods, too. I went in and it was no big deal at all. I kept waiting for it to hurt.

—32C, AGE 46

I got my first mammogram at twenty-five. My mom had just been diagnosed with breast cancer, and my doctor thought I should get checked right away, just to be sure. I had heard the horror stories about how the plates of ice-cold metal squish your breasts into tortillas. I was still in shock from my mom's diagnosis and was worried about whether they would find any cancer in me. I found myself anxious and curious to hurry up and experience my first mammogram. I thought the whole process was fascinating, and I still don't really know how it works, but fortunately they didn't detect any breast cancer.

—36A, AGE 39

Taking care of your breast health is both about what you put on them, like lotions or bras, and what you put into your body, either through diet or exercise. It can also involve what you think about your breasts, especially if your mother, or other close female relative, has had breast cancer. You may be concerned about your own risk of developing breast cancer and would like to consider any preventative measures. Looking at lifestyle choices alone isn't all you can do to ensure your best breast health. You can also get to know your girls, map their unique topography, and introduce them to professional breast screenings, when appropriate. As you grow older, boob checks should be part of your regular health routine. Getting a mammogram doesn't have to be any more inconvenient than a visit to the gynecologist or dentist.

Retail therapy can be a component of breast health, too. Regular bra fittings provide immediate boob-boosting results, ensuring that your girls are getting the support they need. Pampering your silky mounds is important, too. Applying lotions that protect and keep your skin soft, smooth, and unblemished adds to your overall breast maintenance. No product can firm up your breast skin, but if you want to reduce the effects of sun damage and aging, it may be worth your time and effort. Review the muscle groups described in this chapter, and consider starting a program to build up those that can complement the look of your breasts. If nothing else, a well-toned body will add another lovely dimension to your décolleté.

BASIC BREAST CARE

*I never realized until it happened that dry cold weather could
make my breasts itch. Then I would scratch them, thus irritating
and aggravating the problem. Now I moisturize regularly.*

—38C, AGE 33

The most important gift you can give your girls is to watch out for
their best interests. Take a moment to look in the mirror and admire
their wonders. Check out the color and texture of your areolae,
together with the unique dimensions of your nipples. Look at the way
they drop from your chest wall and how these curves look depending
on the angles. No other breasts look or feel exactly like your pair. Be
sure to make more thorough inspections as well, either when you're in
the shower, bath, or lying in bed. If you're not accustomed to doing
breast self-exams (BSEs), start by getting to know your girls and what
they feel like during different times of the month (see appendix for
BSE directions.) Use the Boob Log in the appendix to mark what
you find and keep a record of their changes. Take note of any moles
or other skin lesions that may be of concern. It will serve as your own
record of the ever-changing topography of your breasts.

EXTERIOR MAINTENANCE

SENSIBLE SKIN PROTECTION

Dermatologist and author Dr. Brandith Irwin advises that women
stay away from certain soaps and harsh cleansers around the neck and
chest area. The skin there does need extra attention, but it should be
in the form of moisturizers and sunscreen. "Unless you're in a turtle-
neck, you should put moisturizer and sunscreen on your neck and
chest every morning, just like your face," advises Dr. Irwin. Don't
worry, there's no need to go out and buy any fancy products. If you

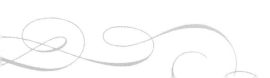

have sensitive skin, you should look for fragrance-free products. Many woman use noncomedogenic (non-pore-clogging) lotions if they have oily skin.

Tanning beds and sun lamps also damage our skin, causing not only skin melanomas (cancers) but premature aging. Even if your skin looks great today, damage from continued unprotected exposure to UV rays (ultraviolet radiation) adds up. Both UVA and UVB rays have been linked to skin cancer.[1] Too much sun can be especially harmful to the thinner skin on your neck and chest. Many dermatologists recommend wearing a sunscreen with an SPF of 30 or higher.

ECZEMA
Sometimes areolae and nipples will develop red patches of itchy, scaly skin. Usually both nipples are affected. Eczema is usually treated with hydrocortisone cream.[2]

NIPPLE HAIR
Many women have one or two stray nipple hairs, while some gals have more than they prefer. You can tweeze them, shave them off,

or use depilatory (hair removal) creams, although all those options could cause some skin irritation. To obtain more-permanent results, consider laser hair removal.

ZITS ON TITS AND OTHER ANOMALIES

Women may experience breakouts on and around their breasts, especially if they participate in regular athletic activities that involve sweating and sports bras. Dr. Irwin recommends using an over-the-counter benzoyl peroxide treatment or a mild hydrocortisone cream. Wearing the wrong-size or ill-fitting sports bra can also cause skin eruptions and rashes. Moisture-wicking fabrics keep you dry and help your skin breathe. Professional triathletes and cyclists also use anti-chafing creams to reduce problems associated with vigorous sports. If you have sensitive skin, another irritant to be aware of is metal, particularly nickel, which is found in many bras and known to be a skin allergen. If you start noticing any skin irritations, check to make sure that your hooks and fasteners aren't the culprits before you try a topical cream.

Women whose boobs grew rapidly in puberty, or during pregnancy and childbirth, may find stretch marks on their skin. While many products on the market claim to prevent or reduce their appearance, how they look has more to do with genetics than the results of any product. The good news is that most stretch marks fade over time and become much less noticeable.

Cracked nipples can be painful and problematic for many pregnant women. Pure lanolin is helpful for some women, but it can cause further irritation in those with allergies to wool. Dr. Irwin recommends considering olive oil or shea butter as alternatives.

If anything more unusual than stretch marks or dry skin appears on or around your breasts, make sure to consult a dermatologist right away. Any excess itching or bleeding—or anything that appears suddenly—should be checked out by a professional.

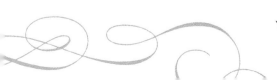

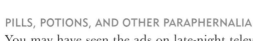

PILLS, POTIONS, AND OTHER PARAPHERNALIA

You may have seen the ads on late-night television or Internet pop-ups claiming that one pill or another potion will magically make your breasts larger or perkier. The truth is that the only pill that enhances breasts temporarily is the birth control pill, and that's mostly caused by increased water retention. Herbal remedies and other lotions claiming to increase or firm your breasts may contain the hormone estrogen, but the quantities used are so minuscule that it would be impossible for them to have any effect. There is no evidence that any of these products live up to their promises.[3]

The one non-FDA-approved system on the market that has received positive comments from users is the Brava Breast Enhancement and Shaping System. Its website states that the device (two suctionlike cups placed on the breasts) must be worn ten hours a day for ten to sixteen weeks to achieve results. They claim that women can increase their breast size from one-half to two cup sizes with consistent use of its product.[4] Another Internet site, Brav-argh! (not affiliated with Brava), provides a forum and blog, complete with comments and advice from other users. Some women claim modest breast enhancement (up to one cup size) but others complain about rashes, irritations, and skin problems associated with the suctioning system, whether properly used or not.[5] Doctors have expressed concern that there have been no long-term studies done of this device, especially with regard to whether increasing breast tissue mass in this manner is safe.[6]

The only known ways to reduce breast size are through surgery or weight loss. Diet and exercise won't allow you to control the amount of fat you want to lose in your breasts, though. You'll be losing weight everywhere else at the same time. Surgical breast reduction appears to be the best option for women who wish to lessen their breast burden. If you choose this route, you will have to trade some scars for smaller breasts. You might also have to pay

DEVELOPED MUSCLES SUIT YOUR SISTERS

Working each one of the following muscle groups will
add definition and beauty to your upper body.

Chest: pectorals. These muscles rest directly beneath your boobs.
Building them up won't increase your cup size, but will give your girls a
stronger base and may make them appear a bit perkier.

Front, middle, and rear shoulders: deltoids. Toned and strong
shoulders are a must for looking good in your swimsuit or any
sleeveless top, plus they help keep those pesky bra straps in their place.

Front and back of upper arms: biceps and triceps. While not directly
related to keeping up our girls, they do sit on either side of our breasts.
Well-toned arms give us confidence and make us look fit in our
strapless and sleeveless tops.

Upper back: lats (latissimus dorsi), traps (trapezius), and romboids.
One good way to keep back fat at bay is to work your upper back
muscles. A strong back will also improve posture.

Six Tips for Your Tits

Suck In Tummy/Breasts Look Yummy
Stand Up Straight/Girls Feel Great
Pull Back Shoulders/Raise Up Boulders
Build Strong Backs/Boobs Look Stacked
Toned, Firm Arms/Frame Breast Charms
Flexed Pecs/Boost Chests

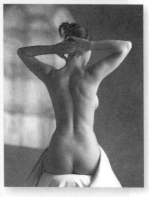

Tony McConnell/Photo Researchers, Inc.

any out-of-pocket costs unless your health insurance covers such procedures. (See Chapter 11: Cut and Paste.)

PHYSICAL FITNESS TIPS FOR YOUR TITS

Maintaining your ideal weight keeps your breasts from going up and down the bra cup scale. Everyone knows that regular exercise and eating a balanced diet (including drinking plenty of water) controls weight gain, but adding weight-bearing exercises can improve the shelf on which your breasts rest.

Posture plays a critical role in helping your girls sit high and pretty. Too often, bosomy gals believe that if they roll their shoulders in, it will make their breasts appear smaller. This forces their bodies to bend down and forward, which literally lowers their boob profile. If you suffer from neck or shoulder pain, bad posture will make those conditions worse. Fitness and wellness expert Shirley Archer asserts, "Posture is the key to both beauty and health. Standing properly makes you appear more confident, slimmer, and taller—and some experts estimate as much as five pounds slimmer and an inch taller."[7] Another terrific way to improve your posture is by doing Pilates or yoga. And your girls won't be the only part of your body that benefits from this type of strength-training exercise.

BREAST EMBELLISHMENTS

Perhaps you've considered adding something more permanent to the landscape of your breasts, either through tattooing or nipple piercing. One note of caution: Any time you break the skin on your body, you introduce the risk of possible infection. Before you decide on any procedure, shop around and make sure you choose a reputable and professional body artist.

TIT TATTOOS

Breast tattoos are common. One major consideration is the choice
of design. If you think your breasts might be less perky in the future
(whether because of weight gain during pregnancy or family history),
you may want to think about how your tattoo could look after your
skin stretches. Many women who have had mastectomies opt to tattoo
the area around the scar rather than undergo breast reconstruction.
Other women get tattoos on their rebuilt breasts, either as part of
the process of replicating a nipple where there isn't one anymore, or
as a decorative embellishment reflective of a woman's personal style.
Some women, especially those who have had breast lumpectomies,
may have heard that tattoos and MRI (Magnetic Resonance Imaging) don't mix. This is reportedly due to higher levels of iron oxide
found in some tattoo inks, which could result in a burning sensation
around the tattoo area when exposed to the magnetic fields that are
part of MRI technology. Radiologists at Seattle Cancer Care Alliance
monitor patients with tattoos and have not discovered any increased
discomfort in this patient population.

NIP PIERCINGS

Nipple piercing is a popular choice among men and women alike.
Again, researching a reputable professional to perform your piercing

will help reduce the risk of possible infection. Some other problems include developing an allergy to the metal in the jewelry. However, nipple piercings do not hinder a woman's ability to breastfeed, unless the piercing was done improperly and damages milk duct tissue. It can take your body longer to recover from having your nipples pierced than certain other body parts, anywhere from three to six months, or more. It's generally recommended that you remove nipple rings while you breastfeed, as they might interfere with latching or be a choking hazard for your baby.[8]

INTERIOR CONSIDERATIONS

Sometimes the only way to tell what's going on inside your breasts is through the art of tactile communication. In other words, you need to become intimate with your own pair. Even if you've made an effort to get to know your own breasts, you may not have a clue as to whether how they feel is how they should feel. And unless a woman's sexual orientation has given her some bonus boob knowledge, her own breasts are very likely the only ones she's ever touched. It's no wonder some of us may be frightened of what lies beneath. Many of these fears can be lessened or eliminated by learning more about breast composition and cancer risk and by monitoring our own overall health.

BREAST CANCER: INCIDENCE AND RISK

The two strongest risk factors for developing breast cancer are being a woman and getting older.
—ANNE MCTIERNAN, MD; JULIE GRALOW, MD; AND LISA TALBOTT, *BREAST FITNESS*[9]

Women today may be more concerned about their risk of breast cancer than generations past because many more cases are being diagnosed today than forty or fifty years ago. Breast cancer rates rose 30 to

PROBABILITY OF DEVELOPING BREAST CANCER BY AGE[10]

If current age is:	Probability:
20	1 in 1,985
30	1 in 229
40	1 in 68
50	1 in 37
60	1 in 26
70	1 in 24
Lifetime risk:	1 in 8

TOP TEN CAUSES OF DEATH IN U.S. WOMEN[11]

Cause	Number of Deaths
Heart disease	348,986
Cerebrovascular disease	96,262
Lung cancer	68,084
Chronic lower respiratory disease	65,668
Alzheimer's disease	45,122
Breast cancer	41,619
Diabetes	38,781
Accidents	38,739
Influenza and pneumonia	36,384
Colorectal cancer	27,793

40 percent between the 1970s and the 1990s, with the biggest increases measured in women over fifty. Women in North America and Northern European countries have the highest incidence of breast cancer but also the lowest number of deaths from the disease.[12]

For women, the greatest risk factor for breast cancer is aging. In the United States, the average age for diagnosis is sixty-one;[13] 78 percent of invasive breast cancer cases are diagnosed in women fifty or older.[14]

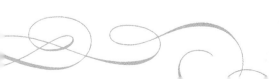

Less than 13 percent of breast cancers are found in women under age forty-four.[15] Around 5 to 10 percent of all breast cancers are thought to be hereditary. Although breast cancer is less common in women under age forty, some doctors think it is more aggressive and less treatable than those types found in older women.[16]

Other factors found to increase a woman's risk include:

- family history of breast cancer (one or more female relatives)
- early menstrual periods (before age twelve)
- not having children or having them after age thirty
- late menopause (age fifty-five+)
- postmenopausal weight gain
- use of hormone replacement therapy (HRT)
- high-density breast tissue
- previous high dose radiation to the chest area
- consuming one or more alcoholic drinks per day

Studies also show that maintaining a healthy body weight, exercising, and breastfeeding may reduce a woman's risk of breast cancer.[17]

DENSE BREASTS ARE NOT DUMB BOOBIES

Many women find out that they have dense breasts when they go in for routine examinations. This means they have a greater proportion of non-fatty breast tissue (which looks more "dense" on a mammogram) compared to fat. One of the reasons that mammography is not recommended for women under age forty is that younger breasts contain more dense tissue. While dense breasts can be more difficult to read for imaging purposes, as we get older, they also carry a higher risk of developing breast cancer.[18]

bOOb*flash!*

NOT IN THE FAMILY

Eighty percent of all women diagnosed with breast cancer have no family history of the disease.[19]

Researchers know that many breast cancers are hormone sensitive, especially to estrogen. Scientists don't understand the exact mechanism but know that estrogen plays some kind of role in the development and growth of breast cancer.[20] While estrogen does not cause cancer by itself, the more of this hormone that women are exposed to during their lifetime, the greater the chance that estrogen may help promote the growth of an estrogen-receptive breast cancer tumor.[21] If we take already estrogen-rich environments (women's bodies) and expose them to additional estrogen, we could increase our risk of developing breast cancers. This may be why breast cancer incidence is higher in Western countries, where women begin menstruating earlier (due to better nutrition), put off childbearing until later, have fewer births, and put off peri- and menopausal symptoms with HRT. "In the 1700s, a forty-year-old woman's life was less estrogen-rich than it is today," says Dr. Constance Lehman. "Women had children at a younger age, breast-fed longer, and usually died of some other disease before even reaching menopause."[22] No one knows exactly to what degree such factors influence a woman's risk of getting breast cancer. Even women with a genetic marker for the disease may never contract it in their lifetime.

Other researchers believe that pollutants and other environmental carcinogens have increased the rates of breast cancer in the United States and other developed countries, and some pesticides are thought to be linked to higher rates of disease in certain populations.[23] Studies also show some association between smoking, and exposure to secondhand smoke, and increased rates of breast cancer.[24] Other factors that have never been shown to cause breast cancer include underwire bras, deodorants and antiperspirants, abortion, and breast implants. For more information about specific studies on breast cancer risk, see the Boobliography.

MONITOR YOUR MAMMARIES FOR OPTIMAL BREAST HEALTH

Because I have dense breasts, my doctor wants me to have a mammogram. But, since I'm also young, my insurance company won't pay for it. As a physical therapist, I work with many young lymphedema patients who have had breast cancer. Insurance companies should remove the age restrictions and pay for mammograms as needed.

—32A, AGE 32

A recent survey by the Society for Women's Health Research found that American women are more afraid of developing breast cancer than they are heart disease, even though the latter is more likely to strike them. Breast cancer ranks sixth out of the ten common causes of death among U.S. women (see sidebar). "Women tend to fear breast cancer more than heart disease, which doesn't make sense from a statistical standpoint because the incidence of heart disease is much greater," says Michael Remetz of Yale Medical Center. Although lung cancer kills more women than breast cancer, fear of contracting lung cancer ranked seventh among greatest female fears in the same study.[25] Whether it's due to greater attention paid during Breast Cancer Awareness month in October, or a hypersensitivity to the thought of treatment that has historically involved some breast disfigurement, women's fear of getting breast cancer is not translating into preventative action.

Every major cancer organization recommends some type of recurrent screening mammography for women forty and older. But studies show that nearly 50 percent of women in this age group do not get regular mammograms.[26] Even though no one knows what (exactly) causes breast cancer, one thing is clear: The earlier it is found the more treatment options are available. And mammography detects 85–90 percent of breast cancers in women over fifty up to two years before a tumor might be felt through a self-exam.[28] Studies have also found that regular clinical breast exams (CBEs), a thorough physical and visual exam conducted by a medical professional, may also detect cancers not found through mammography.[29]

Most health agencies advise women to have a clinical breast exam every three years, beginning at the age of twenty, and yearly CBEs and mammograms starting at age forty. Some medical authorities think the breast self-exam (you know, the one most of us avoid every month), has little value because women don't know how to perform them or don't want to do them. The American Cancer Society now views them as optional for women, and even Dr. Susan Love believes they are no more effective than when women casually feel their own breasts.[30] However, nearly 80 percent of all breast lumps big enough to feel are found by women themselves.[31] Of those lumps, approximately 80 percent are determined to be benign (noncancerous).[32]

Everyone's family health history is unique, and you should consult your own physician about the best way to monitor your specific breast health. Your doctor may suggest other methods of keeping your tits in tip-top shape. For instance, women with a strong family history of breast cancer may be advised to have a baseline mammogram taken

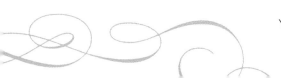

earlier than age forty. (These first mammograms can then be compared to any future images to determine what is normal for your breasts.) The American Cancer Society and many other organizations also recommend annual MRI screening for some high-risk women. And when it comes to your boobs, you can *never* have too much information. Besides, boobs are always changing, so why not take a more hands-on approach to getting to know your girls a little better? (Or enlist the help of a loving partner by indulging in a bit of Boob Foreplay. See section later in this chapter.)

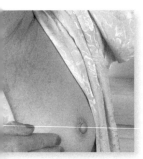

David Davis/Photo Researchers, Inc.

BREAST SELF-EXAM

The BSE is a very specific way to learn about your girls while you are in three separate positions: lying down, standing up, and looking at them in a mirror. It should be performed monthly, around the same time, usually a few days after your period, when any breast tenderness and swelling has subsided. Next time you're at the doctor's, ask for information in order to get a thorough understanding of how to perform your own BSE. You may also want to refer to one of the helpful videos available online or see the directins in the appendix (see also the Boobliography for additional resources). Then record any observations you and/or the doctor find in the Boob Log in the appendix.

Here are some common symptoms associated with breast cancer:

- a lump or any thickening of the breast skin, either on your breast or under your arm
- change in the size or shape of your breast
- nipple discharge or tenderness, or if the nipple suddenly turns inward
- ridges or pitting of the breast (skin looks and has the texture of an orange peel)

► changes to the way breast skin, areola, or nipple look or feel (for example, if any of those areas are warm, swollen, red, or scaly)[33]

CLINICAL BREAST EXAM (CBE)

A CBE is performed by a physician or other health professional, usually at an annual checkup. Most women receive one when they go in for a pap smear or regular physical exam. While lying down, the doctor will examine your entire breast tissue, from collarbone to the area under your arms, and your nipples for any discharge. CBEs are important because (a) not all breast cancers show up on mammograms, and (b) they're an effective detection tool for women who have not yet had a mammogram or who have no access to imaging facilities. The American Cancer Society recommends that every woman over twenty have a CBE every three years and every woman over forty have one annually.

MAMMOGRAM

A mammogram is an FDA-approved, low-dose x-ray of the breast. There are two types of mammograms currently in use: digital and film. Most women won't notice any difference between the two. Both involve the same kind of machine that flattens the breast like a pancake between two plastic or metal shelves. Regular film mammography is done by a radiologist who reads the actual picture against a light box (like a typical x-ray). Digital mammography allows the image to be displayed on a computer screen, which can then be enlarged if there are any areas of interest. Both screening processes work great for normal boob owners, although recent studies show that digital mammography may be more useful in women who have dense breasts, are perimenopausal, or are under the age of fifty.[34] Since it's a newer and more expensive technique, digital mammography is only available at about 8 percent of all facilities.

Mammograms are fairly simple and take about twenty minutes to

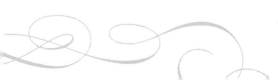

perform. You will be asked to undress from the waist up and to put on a front-closing dressing gown. A technician will take you into a room with the equipment. You will be asked to remove one side of your gown and to place your breast on the shelf of the machine. The technician may have to make some adjustments to ensure that as much tissue as possible will be viewed. Then the upper part of the machine is lowered onto your breast and it is flattened as much as possible. Two views are usually taken of each breast. Some women may find mammograms an uncomfortable experience, or worse, while others seem not to have any particular problem with the procedure. It's best to try to schedule your mammogram during a time of the month when your breasts aren't overly sensitive.

If you have dense breasts, they may be more difficult to read, and you may be called back in to have a second mammogram. Since about 40 percent of all women have dense breasts, this is not unusual, and there's no reason to be alarmed.[37] By law, all mammogram facilities must provide you with written results within thirty days. Most will contact you within five working days if they find any problem or have a concern.[38]

MAMMOGRAM MYTH-INFORMATION

Recommendations for breast mammography may seem as confusing as the different methods used to measure our boobs for a bra. One group of physicians might state that all women should have regular mammograms beginning at age forty, while another association will say it isn't necessary. You will have to decide for yourself what makes sense for your own breast interests. You may want to keep the following in mind when making your decision: (1) Studies show that radiation risk from mammography is negligible and not likely to increase your risk of breast cancer,[39] and (2) mammography is currently the only cost-effective way to detect most—but not all—breast cancers in their early stages. Until researchers can come up with some other method, this is one of the best ways to keep an eye on our inner breast health.

Other imaging techniques that may be employed, but only if something unusual needs to be studied further or if you have a strong family history of breast or ovarian cancers, are ultrasound and MRI. Neither of these involve any radiation and have been shown to be less invasive than performing a physical biopsy of the breast. Some studies have shown that in younger women with a very high risk of breast cancer, MRI may be more helpful in finding their particular cancers.[40] The American Cancer Society now recommends that women with certain high-risk factors for breast cancer have both a yearly mammogram and an MRI.

Including the above detection measures as part of your normal health regimen doesn't prevent breast cancer, but it can help find it

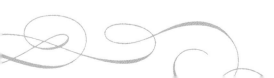

at its earliest possible stage. Early detection has not only been shown to save lives (since the sooner you are able to treat this disease, the better chance of survival), it also means you may have more treatment options. Since the majority of breast lumps are benign, it makes the breast sense to schedule an appointment with your doctor if you find anything out of the ordinary.

PUT YOUR BEST BREAST FORWARD

One of the ways you can improve your breast health is to take good care of your heart. Everything from watching what you eat, maintaining your weight, and refraining from (or quitting) smoking will benefit your boobs. In addition to using common sense to lengthen your life, you can also make it a practice to keep an eye out for any changes to your breast topography. Any questions or concerns that come up should be directed to your healthcare provider. If you know your own breasts well, you can better communicate what's normal (or not) to your own physician. Here are a few ways to make boob health a priority:

BOOB FOREPLAY

For whatever reasons, most women do not perform monthly BSEs. It might be that they're just too boring (or clinical). If that's the case, why not make them more interesting? Enlist your partner to provide an extra set of hands. Asking your sweetie to take charge of your monthly breast exam takes the pressure off and provides another regular reminder to get it done. He or she can gently undress your girls and use the chart on the Boob Log to mark any sensitive areas. This could be followed by a moisturizing massage. Even if there isn't someone else you'd put in charge of your boobs, why not make your own play date with your girls every month? Start off in a luxurious bath with scented candles for atmosphere. Take the time to develop an intimate relationship with your girls and better boob health practices.

MAKE A DATE WITH YOUR GIRL(FRIEND)S

Make a point of scheduling your mammograms with one or more friends. It's not only a great way to keep abreast of each other's health, but you'll have someone to laugh with over the unstylish gowns they make you wear or the absurdity of getting your boobs squeezed between two plates. If anyone gets a "call back" (the second exam technicians often need when imaging more-dense breasts), she will have some supportive company during the wait. Afterward, you can dress your breasts at your favorite lingerie store, or celebrate in style at a girls-only lunch. Being good to your girls should be fun and rewarding!

IMPROVING BREAST HEALTH
FOR GALS EVERYWHERE

Eating right, exercising, and keeping a watchful eye over your own girls is a great start to achieving optimal breast health. And you can help advance research and early detection programs for breast cancer by participating in any of the following:

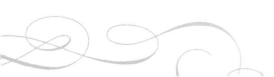

PINK OUT

From ribbons to candy-colored motor scooters, you can buy many different products to benefit breast cancer causes. But buyers also need to be savvy consumers and read the fine print. Some manufacturers of such pink paraphernalia give little back to health organizations. Other people believe that such cause-marketing campaigns spend more in advertising than is ultimately donated to charity.[41] In some cases, you may be better off making a direct contribution to the nonprofit of your choice. For more information, please visit Breast Cancer Action's Think Before You Pink website at www.thinkbefore youpink.org.

WALK, RUN, OR WRITE A CHECK

Many groups hold walks, runs, and even climbs to benefit breast cancer causes. You typically pay a fee to join and gather pledges from friends and associates. Most of these groups provide training and literature on how to succeed. Participanting reaps further rewards in addition to raising dollars, both in bonding with others but also in overcoming many of the physical challenges involved. Look for a list of websites and groups in the Boobliography.

PARTICIPATE IN A CLINICAL TRIAL

According to the National Cancer Institute, clinical trials are important because they test new medical approaches to treating diseases, such as breast cancer. While the majority of cancer trials involve patients who are undergoing treatment for cancer, there are other preventative, screening, and genetic studies that seek participants who have never had cancer. Many different groups, including government agencies, educational institutions, and foundations, sponsor clinical trials all over the world. To learn more about clinical trials, see the Boobliography.

BOTTOM BOOB LINE

No one really knows what causes breast cancer, or why one person with no history or other risk factors finds a malignant lump, while another woman does not. The best we can do is to use the tools currently available for early detection, such as breast exams and mammography. Keeping track of where and when you have any breast problems will provide a solid record of what's normal for your particular boobs. Use the Boob Log in the appendix, which was created for that very purpose. Since you want to live a long and healthy life, be sure to focus on everything you can do to prevent disease, and not just those that impact your breasts. After all, we're much more than just a pair of tits.

CHAPTER TEN

In Sickness and in Health: Coping with Breast Disease and Illness

My mom had breast cancer and ended up getting reconstructive surgery. Her breasts are different now, different shapes, and there are some scars. One implant is tight and hardened. I think she looks beautiful, and I love her newfound confidence with her new breasts!
—34C, AGE 37

Over the years, mine grew to a beautiful B, and they were often seen as perfect to many a man. So it was really hard for me to imagine losing one to cancer. I had an involuntary lumpectomy. But, I got lucky and could keep the nipple and hardly notice now that one is smaller.
—34 (ONE A/ONE B), AGE 34

Just as our breasts are unique, so are breast ailments. Some are benign and are not a threat to our health, while others, like breast cancer, are very serious. How we react varies greatly from woman to woman, and every condition operates differently in each woman's body. Some women get used to having painful premenstrual breasts, or recurring cysts filled with fluid, and don't give it much thought. Another woman might be more anxious, either because of a family history of breast or ovarian cancers (which statistically puts her at greater risk), or just because the thought of anything remotely related to the possibility of breast cancer can be worrisome. Neither woman is right or wrong in her approach to her breast problems. All women benefit from knowing as much as they can about breast illnesses. After all, not every breast problem inevitably leads to breast cancer. And a diagnosis of breast cancer may result in quite simple or very complex treatments. How our bodies react to any illness depends on a host of other variables, from the state of our own health to the severity of our condition.

OUR AILING BREASTS

Oh the joys of cystic breasts. Every year I have a mammogram and every year I spend about an hour being manipulated by the great claw—then a couple of days later I have to return to do it all over again. I have become a pro at staying calm while they figure out if I have breast cancer or not. Cystic breasts are always tender and sometimes they just hurt like crazy.

—36DD, AGE 48

While the prospect of breast cancer provokes fear among women, it's not the only breast illness or other condition we might face. During our breastfeeding years, problems with blocked milk ducts, mastitis, or breast abscesses are likely to crop up. These can be very painful, although temporary, conditions. Women can also suffer from generalized breast pain, known as mastalgia or mastodynia, at any age. Such breast pain can occur during a woman's regular monthly cycle or not be associated with any menstrual or other hormonal fluctuations at all. Half of all women are also diagnosed with "fibrocystic changes" (often referred to as a disease, which it is not) at some point in their lives.[2] Symptoms can include cysts, lumpiness, areas of thickening, tenderness, and pain.

BENIGN BREAST CONDITIONS

The following conditions are often referred to as benign, meaning not cancerous, because they are not thought to increase breast cancer risk. However, any lump, discharge from the nipple, thickening, redness, tenderness, or pain in your breasts should be reported to your physician. Statistically, it's unlikely to be breast cancer, but it is important to get it checked out so you can take the best care of your body. Being proactive about anything that seems unusual will also bring you greater peace of mind and knowledge of what is normal for your individual breasts.

Mastalgia can occur in up to 70 percent of all women.[3] According to Dr. Susan Love, "It can run the gamut of discomfort—from minor irritation a couple of days a month to permanent, nearly disabling agony, and everything in between."[4] Mastalgia usually presents itself in one of two ways. The first is more common and includes symptoms such as swelling, tenderness, general lumpiness, and pain. It comes and goes with our periods and seems related to hormonal changes. The second is more rare and may feel like a stabbing pain or an underlying muscle ache.

Women who suffer from mastalgia should keep a record of the number of days and severity of pain. (Make use of the Boob Log to note this.) Keeping track of the length and intensity of symptoms allows women to see whether their pain is related to cyclical periods and, if not, to report these incidents to their regular physician.

"Most women suffering from mastalgia are much more worried about the possibility that they may have breast cancer than about the pain itself," writes Dr. Miriam Stoppard in *Breast Health*.[5] Women, and even their doctors, may trivialize these types of breast disorders, but it's important for women to get reassurance from a professional if they're worried about breast cancer (which rarely causes this type of pain). That reassurance alone can help resolve the severity of the symptoms in many cases.[6]

Some patients have found relief through prescription medication or making dietary changes, such as cutting back on caffeine, eating a low-fat diet, or taking evening primrose oil (although no definitive studies prove that such remedies work). Not all women respond to the same treatment, so it's important you speak with your own physician about possible solutions. And don't rule out the idea of buying a new bra to solve breast pain. One study of women in Saudi Arabia found that 85 percent of mastaglia sufferers found relief by wearing a good sports bra.[7]

CYSTS

Cysts are small spaces in your breast tissue that fill with fluid and cause pain. A physician will typically confirm that they are benign by draining them with a needle and studying the fluid. Some women have recurring cysts, while others have none or may only have one in their entire lifetime.[8]

FIBROADENOMAS

Benign growths in breast tissue called fibroadenomas usually occur in teens and young women, although they have been found in women going through menopause (and even postmenopausal women who are on hormones). Fibroadenomas are hard and firm, not fluid-filled like cysts, and can show up on mammograms. They may be removed with minimal scarring. Fibroademonas don't always cause pain, but they can be scary because they are lumps and bumps in our breasts. Keep in mind that only a doctor can determine whether they are completely benign.[9]

INTRADUCTAL PAPILLOMA

These are wartlike growths of tissue inside the nipple duct. Intraductal papillomas often cause a bloody discharge, and they're found most often in women between the ages of thirty-five and fifty-five. Treatment involves removal of the area by way of incision on the side of your areola.[10]

MAMMARY DUCT ECTASIA

This ailment is an inflammation of the milk duct that seems to occur in older women, a result of our aging milk ducts. Mammary duct ectasia may result in nipple discharge, and areas of the breast may be tender and red. It is often treated with antibiotics.[11]

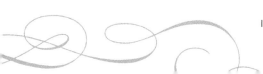

MASTITIS

This condition is usually, but not always, found in women who are breastfeeding, when bacteria find their way into the breast tissue through raw or cracked nipples. Symptoms include pain, swelling, redness, and tenderness and may be accompanied by a fever. This condition is often resolved with antibiotics. In some rarer cases, mastitis may turn into breast abscesses that need to be drained.[12]

BREAST CANCER 101

Being told I had cancer, the one thing I can recall with clarity—despite the shock—is an immediate feeling that I was no longer living on the same planet as the people around me. I had crossed this huge line, and life looked like nothing I had ever seen on the other side. It was almost impossible for me to sit at dinner parties discussing shopping or weekend plans when all I could hear inside my swimmy head was, Shit, you have cancer. *It was as if the rest of my life before the diagnosis took place in the years* BC.

—34B, AGE 34

While it's harder than it should be to find resources on general breast health, there are hundreds of books and web resources covering the topic of breast cancer. Everything you want to know, from dealing with your diagnosis, treatment options, and prevention to personal stories from survivors and families, can be found on the shelves of your local bookstore or at the click of your mouse. Thus, what follows is a general overview of the basics of breast cancer. This chapter introduces you to terms and statistics, and the Boobliography in the appendix lists additional resources for women who need more-detailed information.

So, what is breast cancer? It is the uncontrolled (malignant) growth of cells inside a woman's breasts. "If breast cancer always stayed confined to the breast, it would not be life-threatening," write the authors of *Breast Fitness*, a book on how to reduce your breast cancer risk.[13] The trouble is that these cells can and do move into lymph nodes and blood vessels, traveling to other parts of the body and attacking vital organs. And not all cancer moves at the same speed: Some are slower growing and others are fast. That's why finding breast cancer while it's still localized in our breasts can be crucial for treatment. Attacking the cancer before it's had a chance to metastasize, or spread, is an important factor tied to women overcoming and conquering breast cancer. Yet, it is still not possible for doctors to detect all breast cancers early, any more than women can reduce all risk of developing this disease.

DETECTION

Detection of breast cancer can be a multistep process. You or your doctor may find a lump during an exam, or a mammogram might show an area of calcification, but finding a lump or an irregularity doesn't necessarily result in a cancer diagnosis. More tests need to be done to take a look at your breast tissue from different perspectives. This might include a clinical physical exam, which could be followed by an ultrasound, an MRI, or a biopsy (often used to confirm that a cyst is benign). Some doctors might recommend a different type of procedure, but each is done to make a comprehensive diagnosis. Not all breast cancer presents itself as a "lump," and 80 percent of all lumps are *not* found to be breast cancer.[15]

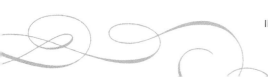

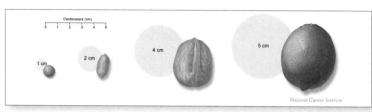

TUMOR SIZES

DIAGNOSIS

A diagnosis of breast cancer can be shocking and difficult to comprehend. After getting this news, many women report going into a trancelike state, unable to understand everything that is being said or done around them. This is compounded by falling boob-first into the cancer world, filled with its own medical terminology and the ins and outs of treatment and recovery. All of a sudden, a woman diagnosed with breast cancer is confronted with overwhelming amounts of information on the multiple kinds of breast cancer, stages, and possible treatment options. A variety of specialists are also needed to meet every aspect of the disease, be they a breast surgeon, oncologist, plastic surgeon (for reconstruction procedures), or physical therapist to recover from cancer treatments.

Breast cancer comes in different forms, which correspond to the variety of places it can rest in your breast (such as the duct, lobe, or general breast tissue). In situ, or "in place," forms are considered precancerous by many physicians, although their presence predicts a higher future risk of a more invasive breast cancer. Some women are diagnosed with more than one type of breast cancer at one time, depending on where it's found. Here are some major (and a few rare but well-known) cancer types:

Lobular carcinoma in situ (LCIS): These are cancerous cells that begin in the lobes of the breast and stay there.

Ductal carcinoma in situ (DCIS): This cancer is usually found through mammography when areas of calcification are present in the breast (which indicates that cancer cells may be active). Like LCIS, this cancer has not spread beyond the duct area. In 2000, DCIS made up 14 percent of all breast cancers diagnosed in the United States.[16]

Invasive or infiltrating ductal carcinoma: This is the most common form of breast cancer, representing around 80 percent of all cases. The cancer has broken through duct walls and invades the breast's fatty tissue. It may then be able to spread to other parts of the body either through the lymphatic system or the bloodstream.

Invasive or infiltrating lobular cancer: This cancer begins in the lobules, but is more spread out in the breast tissue, so it's not as easy to detect as invasive ductal carcinoma. Also, this type has potential to move to other areas of the body.

Paget's disease: A far less common kind of breast cancer, representing 3 percent of all cases, Paget's is thought to begin in the breast ducts and move into the areola and nipple. Symptoms can be confused with those found in eczema of the breasts because skin can be itchy and dry.

Inflammatory breast cancer (IBC): IBC is another rare but aggressive breast cancer, representing about 1 percent of all breast cancers. This cancer makes the breast red, warm, and generally inflamed. You may not have a lump, but your entire breast could be firm and swollen.

Breast cancer is further identified by "stage," meaning how far it has spread to nearby tissue, lymph nodes, or other body organs. This will help doctors determine the prognosis and treatment. In situ cancers are referred to as stage O. Stage I and stage II are considered early-stage cancers with some lymph node involvement. Stage III includes more-advanced cancers, with larger tumors and nodes and possibly some tissue involvement. (For instance, IBC is categorized as a stage III cancer.) Stage IV (metastatic) breast cancer is usually considered incurable, since it has spread further and may be found in the liver, lungs, bones, and elsewhere.[17]

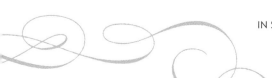

Advances in breast cancer research include targeting specific gene characteristics in order to block tumor growth. One such approach is based on whether the cancer is estrogen or progesterone receptive, growing more quickly when exposed to those hormones, and uses agents that target those receptors directly. Certain therapies, such as tamoxifen (Nolvadex®), may be able to slow tumor growth down. Another marker, called a HER2 protein, has also been found to speed up cancer's cell-replicating process. Drugs such as trastuzumab (Herpecin®) target the HER2 protein. Scientists hope that in the near future treatment can be individualized for each woman's specific breast cancer, avoiding the need to include treatments that may not be as effective.

DECISION

By the time a decision is reached, a woman may have met with several doctors, including a breast surgeon and an oncologist. Some women seek out second and even third opinions. Bombarded with statistics and various scenarios (and even sometimes conflicting information), they may find it difficult to make a decision. In the final analysis, it all depends on the woman's individual situation. If she's younger, she may worry more about any type of recurrence and choose the most aggressive therapy possible. If she's older, and the cancer is thought to be slow growing, she may take a more conservative approach. Whether she has young children at home, or hopes to have more children, is a factor that has to be taken into consideration—not to mention family history or any other medical issues that may come into play. Some women are all alone in their decision, without a partner or supportive friends nearby. There can be concerns about time taken off work, or about insurance coverage. Some women must travel farther for treatment or follow-up observation. For many women (and their families), such choices are made easier by educating themselves about all the alternatives and relying on healthcare providers they

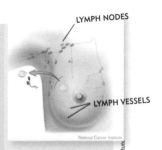

LYMPH NODES

LYMPH VESSELS

National Cancer Institute

CHECKING YOUR NODES

The lymphatic system is part of our body's immune system. It carries "lymph" fluid that filters out bacteria and recycles it back into our bodies. Lymph nodes are where the white cells do battle with anything toxic, which is why they may be swollen when we are fighting some types of infection. Since cancer cells can spread by traveling through our lymph system or our bloodstream, it is important for your doctors to determine whether lymph nodes near breast tissue contain cancer cells.

trust. One breast cancer patient put it this way, "I wanted someone who made me feel like a person and not a statistic. I chose a doctor who treated me that way."

BREAST CANCER TREATMENTS

Only forty years ago, when a breast lump was discovered, a woman would be immediately scheduled for surgery. She would go under anesthesia not knowing whether she'd awaken with her breast(s) still intact. A woman would sign a consent form as part of what was then called a "one-step" procedure. The doctor would cut out the tumor, do an immediate biopsy, and if the results showed cancer, perform a radical mastectomy. Women woke up to both their diagnosis and their treatment decisions having been made for them. The radical mastectomy was performed no matter the size of the tumor or its possible progression, leaving women feeling butchered and very much out of control regarding decisions about their own bodies. Yet, this treatment was viewed as the only way to save the life of a woman who'd been diagnosed with breast cancer. The topic was rarely discussed, unlike today, when you find numerous articles in magazines, a breast cancer awareness month, and countless support groups to help patients through treatment and recovery. We have made inroads in detecting earlier forms of breast cancer, which result in less-disfiguring treatment than the radical mastectomy.

One of the first cases of breast cancer on record was made by an Egyptian physician some 3,500 years ago who held no hope for his patient's survival.[18] Centuries later, doctors continued to speculate as to the cause of the disease but did attempt to treat it by removing tumors. These early excisions were performed hundreds of years before the advent of anesthesia, yet many women were willing to endure any procedure that might prolong their lives. Such attempts to stop the spread of cancer did not have much success. Because the importance of sterile surgical equipment was not yet recognized, patients often died from infection. As it turned out, the same man who introduced the widespread use of surgical gloves was also the man who popularized the radical mastectomy as the best treatment option for women whose breast tumors were found to be cancerous. In the early 1900s, Dr. William Halsted concluded that the radical mastectomy was the best way to prevent a woman from dying from the disease. The procedure involved removing as much of the infected breast tissue and surrounding pectoral muscle as possible, and it became the preferred method for treating breast cancer for the next hundred years.[19]

It wasn't until the mid-1980s, when studies showed that less-extensive removal of tissue by lumpectomy or modified mastectomy was as safe and effective in terms of overall survival rates, that the radical mastectomy fell out of favor as the preferred treatment method. This was not the only factor that led to the decline of the radical mastectomy, however.[20] It was also due to the efforts of many brave women who opposed the one-step procedure and worked hard to ensure that women were allowed to make their own treatment decisions. This campaign to raise awareness brought breast cancer out of the shadows and into the public eye. High-profile women, including Betty Ford, Betty Rollin, and Rose Kushner, were among the many who publicized their own battles with breast cancer and treatment. Breast reconstruction became available in the mid-1970s with new surgical innovations and the advent of breast implants.[21] Yet, it wasn't until 1998 that legislation was enacted to require insurance companies to cover the cost of prostheses and reconstruction after mastectomy.[22] Today, researchers continue to fine-tune treatment methods for every individual woman. Scientists are studying other ways that women can work to reduce their own risk (see Chapter 9: Your Breast Potential). And while there is no known way to prevent the disease, early detection and treatment has resulted in fewer deaths from breast cancer.

WHERE TREATMENT IS TODAY

Today, women have more than the one option of radical mastectomy when it comes to breast cancer treatment. But the type and stage at which breast cancer is diagnosed determines which methods can be used. Most treatments involve some degree of surgery to remove the cancer, followed by nonsurgical methods to keep the cancer from spreading or recurring. Each woman's treatment will be different and her experience with breast cancer unique.

MASTECTOMY

There are various types of mastectomy procedures. Some are "skin sparing," which means that extra skin is left intact for anticipated reconstruction. Most mastectomies involve removing all the breast tissue, including the nipple and some specific lymph nodes, but retaining the major pectoral muscle. Some women with known genetic markers for breast cancer may choose to undergo "prophylactic mastectomy," which entails having both breasts removed to lower their risk of contracting breast cancer in one or both breasts.

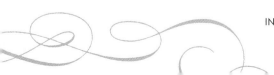

LUMPECTOMY

Also called "breast-conserving surgery," a lumpectomy removes only the specific tissue and skin around the area where the tumor is located.

QUADRANTECTOMY

A quadrantectomy is similar to a lumpectomy except that it involves the removal of more tissue. A quadrantectomy excises around one-quarter of the breast tissue.

CHEMOTHERAPY

Chemotherapy is a drug treatment that can either be taken orally or injected into a specific area of the body to destroy or slow down cancer cells. The quantity and duration of chemotherapy depends on the type and stage of the cancer. Side effects of chemo are numerous and may include hair loss, nausea, fatigue, joint pain, and possible loss of fertility. Despite these drawbacks, chemo has been proven to be very effective in preventing cancer cells from returning.

RADIATION

Radiation is a targeted therapy treatment that focuses on attacking specific areas of the breast to eradicate cancer cells.

HORMONE THERAPY

Taken in the form of a pill, hormone therapies can slow down the ability of cancer cells to replicate. Tamoxifen (Nolvadex®) is one such drug that's shown to be effective in specific cases, although it's not without side effects. There are many hormone therapies that are currently being developed and tested in the ongoing search for better cancer treatments. (See the Boobliography for more information.)

LIFE AFTER TREATMENT

Once a woman has been diagnosed with breast cancer, she is automatically at greater risk of contracting the disease again. Individual risk of recurrence is something every woman needs to discuss with her doctor because it is based on the specifics of the type of cancer diagnosis, where it was found, and how it was treated. Survival rates are highest, 98 percent, for women diagnosed with earlier forms of breast cancer, such as in situ cancers.[23]

Immediate adjustments to lifestyle after treatment include recuperating from surgery, scheduling and going through follow-up treatments, and dealing with side effects. Returning for mammograms and ultrasounds on a regular basis may make women anxious, especially in the aftermath of surgery. Many breast cancer survivors find that joining a support group and/or speaking with other breast cancer survivors is helpful in rebuilding their lives.

About 15 to 20 percent of women who have had their lymph

U.S. BREAST CANCER SURVIVAL RATES

5 years after diagnosis:	88%
10 years:	80%
15 years:	71%
20 years:	63%

According to the American Cancer Society, the most recent information on calculating relative survival rates are based on patients who were diagnosed with breast cancer four to ten years ago. The above statistics do not reflect more-recent changes in detection, treatment, or new drug therapies.[24] Women at a more advanced stage at diagnosis have lower survival rates. The five-year survival rate for those with localized cancer is 98 percent, regional is 83 percent, and distant-stage disease is 26 percent.[25]

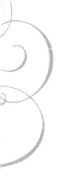

nodes removed or radiated may experience lymphedema, a buildup of lymph fluid that causes painful swelling. This may happen right after surgery or years later and it can last for a few weeks or several months or years.[26] There is no cure for lymphedema, and treatment typically involves physical therapy and the use of compression garments.

SCENARIOS SURROUNDING THE LOSS OF YOUR GIRLS

Not all women choose to undergo reconstruction after breast cancer. Statistics vary, but even after the passage of the law mandating insurance coverage for this procedure, only one out of five women chose to rebuild their breasts.[27] Other studies place the figure closer to two out of every five women.[28] Many women choose not to have reconstructive surgery because they don't want to undergo any additional medical procedure. Some women have reconstruction immediately following their mastectomy, while others choose to wait a while—up to a year or more—to decide what they want to do. Every woman, of course, should choose the option that makes her feel most comfortable.

REMAINING BREAST-FREE
The choice to remain breast-free is made for many individual reasons. Some women are reluctant to have more surgery and prefer the option of prostheses. Others start out using the prosthesis and give it up for a variety of reasons. Other women opt to tattoo the scars left from their mastectomies, embracing the idea of the radical change their bodies have undergone with body art.

CHOOSING BREAST PROSTHESES
Using a breast prosthesis is a good solution for women who have had mastectomies but wish to retain their former silhouette in their clothing. Prostheses can be made to order, exactly to size, and come in various materials.

UNDERGOING BREAST RECONSTRUCTION

For some women, breast reconstruction is closure. They might feel that having their breasts reconstructed will allow them to face a more "normal," or at least normal-looking, life. This is especially true for younger women who may want to continue to wear swimsuits and the latest fashions without having to deal with the limitations posed by prostheses. But reconstruction is nothing like an ordinary boob job. Women with rebuilt breasts will not regain nipple or tissue sensation lost through mastectomy. Depending on the type of cancer and future treatment, reconstruction options may be simple or more complex. Even though they may have had to endure further hospital-ization, time away from work and family, recovery, and additional scarring, many women are pleased with the results of their surgery. (For more information on reconstruction, see Ch. 11, Cut and Paste.)

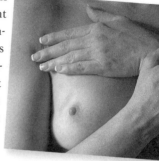

Michele Taras

GATHER INFORMATION

Dealing with any kind of illness in your life can be a traumatic experience. If you've been diagnosed with breast cancer, or know someone who has, the first step is to learn about what you're facing and what your options are. The second is to ensure that you have a good support system to lean on during this difficult time. Lastly, you may decide to reprioritize how you live your life, both to include a possible risk of recurrence and to help lower the incidence of breast cancer for future generations of women. See the Boobliography for organizations, support groups, and websites that are a critical piece of the information-gathering process.

INVESTIGATE AND INQUIRE

Read books, surf the web, or contact other breast cancer survivors to learn more about what you are facing. You may want to limit yourself to resources recommended by friends, family, and physicians in order to avoid becoming overwhelmed by the large amount of (sometimes conflicting) information that's available. If you feel the need, seek second or third medical opinions, and be prepared for the work involved in finding your own breast surgeon, oncologist, plastic surgeon, and other practitioners. Speak up and assert yourself. Make sure all your questions are thoroughly answered, even if it is medically impossible to predict the future.

CREATE YOUR OWN SUPPORT STRUCTURE

Patients often find it easier to join support groups, not only to connect with others who can share your new circumstances, but also to hear from women who are long-term survivors. Talking to other women about their experiences may help to allay your fears.

SHARE THE CHALLENGE

Rotate duties among friends and family. Many people will be anxious to help but may not know how to ask or what they can do. Consider sending email updates on your progress, letting the people you love know if you need help with kids, meals, or trips to the grocery store. You can also consider sharing the names of websites where your friends and family can get tips on how to provide support.

TAKE ACTION TOWARD PREVENTION

Once you're through with your therapy, you may want to take a closer look at your lifestyle and assess any additional risk factors you have for the disease. Beyond that you may want to join organizations focused on reducing possible cancer-causing agents in our environment. While millions of dollars have been spent on breast cancer

bOOb*flash!*

COLOR CONTRASTS

Breast cancer rates are highest among white women over the age of thirty-five. Among women under age thirty-five, African American women have a slightly higher incidence than white women, and they're more likely to die from breast cancer at any age.[29] In 2002, African American women experienced a 37 percent higher death rate from breast cancer than white women.[30] Incidence and death rates from breast cancer are lower among all other ethnic and racial groups.

detection and treatment, there are many other groups dedicated to eradicating the disease through research.

LOOK AT THE FUTURE

Having any kind of breast illness is scary. Our breasts sit on our chest, conveniently located in a place that is visible to us and others. The thought that we might miss a warning sign, or have a higher risk of contracting cancer because we put off having children or did not breastfeed, may contribute to feelings of regret or guilt. But one risk factor may be reduced by another, and no one can say how much any of these factors have to do with contracting breast cancer. After all, even women who carry a much greater genetic risk may never develop the disease. While breast cancer is the second most diagnosed cancer among women worldwide (after skin cancers), it also has one of the highest survival rates—especially if diagnosed early. New drug therapies, together with less-disfiguring treatments, do not make facing this disease an easy task, but they do offer hope.

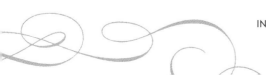

CHAPTER ELEVEN

Cut and Paste: Surgical Answers to Breast Dilemmas

My dad tells the story of the time he was giving me a bath when I was three, and I looked down at my chest, tapped my nipples, and asked, "When am I going to get bumples, like Mommy?" Apparently he said something like "Be patient," or "Someday." But it was all a lie. I finally had to go out and buy some!
—34C, AGE 35

I had a reduction. Loved the results but wish they were a little smaller. The doctor was good, kept all natural feeling intact. My husband likes the loss of inhibition that my modesty about my bigger breasts brought out in me.
—FORMERLY 36DD, NOW 34C/D, AGE 46

You hear talk around the watercooler that Sheila in accounting had a boob job. Does that mean she had implants? Maybe . . . or maybe not. Once used only to refer to breasts made bigger through silicone or saline implants, today a "boob job" could mean any number of cosmetic or restorative breast surgeries. A woman might choose to have her breasts made smaller by undergoing a breast reduction, or made perkier with a breast lift. Another may go for implants, not just to make her bosom bigger, but to get back the volume she may have lost through pregnancy and nursing. A woman who chooses to have a breast augmentation (the technical term for breast implant surgery) won't necessarily have noticeably bigger breasts, either. Your own mother might have had a boob job, but unless you've seen her nude boobs, you may never know.

Just as bras can help reshape saggy, small, or too-big breasts, so can going under the knife. Cosmetic surgery is another way to change our breast appearance, although not everyone agrees that going to these lengths to alter your girls is a good idea. But breast surgeries are becoming increasingly popular, whether to reduce, increase, lift, reconstruct, or even correct breast defects. You can even change the size and shape of your areolae or nipples. Yup, all of these procedures are available—for a price. And all involve varying degrees of risk, which must be weighed against any physical and/or psychological rewards.

There are pros and cons to any type of surgery. One way to make an informed decision is to arm yourself with as much information as possible. While many different types of procedures exist, results vary from woman to woman. Again, your individual breasts come into play, along with your medical history and concerns for your future health. Understanding the history of certain cosmetic breast procedures puts into perspective why there is still so much controversy over silicone implants, for instance. An informational consult with an experienced plastic surgeon is a must before undergoing serious surgery: It will expand your knowledge and help predict your individual results. Living with your new breast self is another aspect of breast surgery you may not have thought about. Once you go under the knife, you can't go back.

MAN(RE)MADE BOOBS

The word "plastic" in plastic surgery doesn't refer to some artificial material. It comes from the Greek word *plastikos,* meaning to shape or mold. These types of surgeries have been performed for thousands of years, getting their start in ancient India. The first recorded breast reduction was performed on a man in 625 AD.[1] It wasn't until 1895 that surgery was first attempted to correct a woman's asymmetrical breasts.[2] Before the advent of anesthesia or antibiotics, these surgeries weren't too popular. When doctors developed techniques to treat wounded soldiers during World War I, reconstructive plastic surgery advanced significantly. Since that time, it has been one of the fastest-growing medical fields.[3]

Whether to improve one's looks cosmetically, or as a means to repair or restore a physical defect due to accident, disease, or genetics, plastic surgery is here to stay. This is evidenced by the number of women and men willing to go under the knife each year and surveys of our own attitudes about such surgeries. Public opinion polls show that more than 55 percent of women and 52 percent of all men in the United States approve of cosmetic surgery.[4] Another survey found that while only 6 percent of the adult population has had a cosmetic surgery procedure, almost 20 percent plan to at some point in their lives. And it's not the pain of surgery that postpones their decision making; it's the cost. But many of these enthusiasts are reluctant to cop to their openness about future procedures: Only 33 percent said they would admit to it when asked.[5]

Plastic surgery is divided into two subgroups: cosmetic, which is considered "elective" and is not covered by insurance, and reconstructive, which is performed to restore some part of the body that's

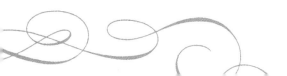

TOP FIVE FEMALE AND MALE SURGICAL COSMETIC PROCEDURES FOR 2006[6]

Female	Male
Breast augmentation 329,999	Nose reshaping 85,000
Liposuction 268,000	Eyelid surgery 37,000
Nose reshaping 223,000	Liposuction 35,000
Eyelid surgery 196,000	Hair transplantation 20,000
Tummy tuck 140,000	Male breast reduction 20,000

been altered by disease or congenital defect and is thus viewed as medically necessary. In 2006, there were more than 1.8 million cosmetic surgical procedures performed in the United States. Of those 329,000 were breast augmentations and 104,000 breast lifts. In the reconstruction category, by comparison, women underwent 104,000 breast reductions and 56,000 breast reconstructions.[7] In 2006, women made up 90 percent of the U.S. cosmetic surgery patient population; however, among men who do opt for plastic surgery, boob-related procedures (specifically breast reduction for gynecomastia[8]) were the fifth most common type of surgery.[9]

Cosmetic surgery can be taken to extremes, as seen in popular reality TV shows like *Extreme Makeover* and *The Swan*. Plastic surgeons Dr. Allen Rosen and Dr. Valerie Ablaza, authors of *Beauty in Balance,* write in their book that these programs "foster the myth that plastic surgery is a quick and easy fix."[10] Most people don't—and shouldn't—undergo multiple medically complicated procedures to change everything about themselves over such a short period of time. But there are those willing to do so, possibly because they're obsessed or dissatisfied with their appearance. They may suffer from body dysmorphic disorder (BBD), an illness that's thought to be caused by a chemical imbalance in the brain. Some 15 percent of patients undergoing cosmetic surgery suffer from this debilitating disorder.[11] Their symptoms can often be made worse by plastic surgery, and many psychologists recommend that people with BDD be treated with therapy and antidepressants rather than indulging their condition with more frequent, costly, and often risky procedures.[12] Most surgeons agree that the best plastic surgery candidates are people who possess a positive self-image and realistic expectations.

THE POLITICALLY INCORRECT BREAST

I haven't had breast reduction, but it's something I'm considering. I don't know what people's reaction would be, especially as I'm deeply feminist. Some people would see it as a betrayal in the fight against body fascism. But those people aren't suffering the back pain, discomfort, and body dysmorphia that big breasts can cause.

—32FF, AGE 31

Despite the fact that public opinion polls show that plastic surgery is more accepted than ever before, there's still a not-so-subtle prejudice against women who choose to surgically alter their breast shape and size. This notion may reflect the enormous power boobs wield in our society. We can always choose to falsely advertise artificially larger or firmer breasts with the help of a bra, but go under the knife to achieve the same result? For some, that's simply going too far. Messing with our mammaries, especially if it involves augmentation, is often criticized. Websites like Tit 4 Tat "stomp on breast implant hype with the 'no silicone, no saline, no sir!' attitude" and sell T-shirts and other gear belittling implants.[13] Victoria's Secret model and TV host Tyra Banks became so fed up with implant rumors about her breasts that she had a public breast sonogram on her show just to prove they were "real."[14] The popular sex manual *Guide to Getting It On* states that "women with plastic chests attract men with plastic brains."[15] The author contends that women seeking implants only do so to meet society's preference for a larger breast. Is it true that women have been blinded by

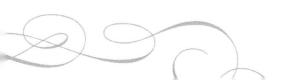

advertisements that are tricking us into believing that bigger is better and that women who seek enhancements do so just to create that look? "I don't care what anyone tells you, huge fake breasts are freaky,"[16] writes a columnist for *Elle* magazine. Books such as *Our Bodies, Ourselves* imply that women who choose implants perpetuate the idea that thin women with big busts are most attractive to men.[17] In fact, there is such a strong negative stereotype associated with women who opt for larger-size breast implants that some doctors warn women that they may be criticized for their choice to go big.[18]

Critics of breast plastic surgeries argue that our society is fixated on women's appearance as a measure of their worth and that the media is responsible for the glorification of unrealistic body types. Many people think that women aren't making unbiased personal choices about plastic surgery because they're bombarded daily by images of unnaturally perky-breasted Victoria's Secret models (except Tyra Banks, of course). Opponents of plastic surgery also point to the increased costs to society resulting from illnesses that crop up in the aftermath of silicone implants gone bad or other botched breast surgeries. Even breast cancer patients have come under fire. When advancements in reconstructive surgery techniques first made the option available, some chastised mastectomy patients for not wearing their scars proudly, as a symbol of survival. Of course, it's important to remember that some people will criticize any choice a woman makes, which is why it's crucial that every woman be entitled to make her own decision.

Alex Kuczynski, author of *The Beauty Junkies,* is another writer who suggests that most women who choose plastic surgery simply want to be viewed as sexually desirable and attractive to the opposite sex,[19] (although no statistics exist with regard to implant patients' sexual preferences). It's true that the female breast is one of the most prominent symbols of sexual lust in our society, which is why a woman who's concerned with her looks may focus on her boobs. And the billion-dollar beauty industry does pull a lot of weight when it comes to influencing our decisions about how we should look.

Some women believe we'd be celebrated more for our hearts and minds than our physical appearance if we stopped doing all the things that are imposed on us by our beauty-conscious culture—whether that's implants, dying our hair, or wearing makeup. But our desire to look good might run deeper than social expectations. Finding other people attractive gives us information—about their health, fertility, and potential as a future mate. "Beauty is not going anywhere," writes Nancy Etcoff in her book *Survival of the Prettiest*. "The idea that beauty is unimportant or a cultural construct is the real beauty myth."[20] Men and women alike understand that being attractive is an asset. An American Cosmetic Surgery poll found that five out of six consumers believe that "personal appearance is key to professional success."[21] Questions of fairness aside, beautiful people get the best jobs, have more sexual partners, and are treated better by others. Studies show that the impact of this "beauty bias" may influence a person's decision to have plastic surgery.[22]

Given all the controversy, you'd expect plastic surgeries to be met with mixed patient results. Yet, in general, cosmetic breast surgeries seem to improve a woman's self-esteem and outlook on life. The happiest cosmetic surgery patients are those who undergo breast surgery (whether it's to make their boobs bigger or smaller). Years after their operations, women report being less depressed, having a higher quality of life, and less stress and anxiety.[23] A 2007 study found that breast augmentations significantly boosted a woman's self-esteem and sexuality.[24]

When people question boob jobs, it's usually the augmentation procedures and lifts that come under scrutiny. It's easier for others to empathize with women who are seeking out breast reductions for relief from too-heavy breasts that may have caused years of shoulder, neck, and back pain. Breast reductions have been performed since the

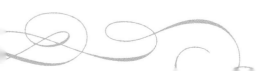

ARE NEW BOOBS FOR YOU?

If you answer yes to any of the following, you may want to reconsider whether plastic surgery is right for you.

I plan to get pregnant in the future. Pregnancy changes your breasts and will definitely alter their size and shape, regardless of surgery.

I want to breastfeed my children. Some surgical procedures make it more difficult, or impossible, to nurse. Review possible complications carefully. You may want to put off surgery until you're done birthing babies.

I'm in poor physical and/or financial health. Any surgery carries some risk, so the better health and shape you are in, the more likely a successful result. You should also feel financially secure, since (a) you will probably pay thousands of dollars out of pocket to cover the cost, and (b) future corrective surgeries should be anticipated.

I have a history of breast cancer in my family. While no studies link an increased risk of breast cancer with implants, they can make mammograms more difficult to read. Ask your doctor whether the kind of breast implant placement you choose will interfere with future breast imaging.

I don't want any scars. Scars are a fact of life with any type of surgery, although you could scar less—or more—than another person.

I'm not willing to trade possible loss of nipple sensation for new boobs. Nipple sensitivity can decrease, or increase, and can be temporary or permanent. No medical professional can guarantee that you'll have the same, more, or less sensitivity.

I want new boobs to please my partner, or attract a mate. Never make a physical change to your body merely to please someone else. If your partner doesn't love you for who you are inside, they'll only be temporarily satisfied with some outward change.

1920s, yet in the 1930s, reductions were often considered "cosmetic" and women who desired the procedure criticized for being vain.[25]

IMPLANT DISCRIMINATION

Nearly three million American women have had breast augmentations since 1980. The average cup size they request is a "full C," but each year a larger percentage of women opt for jumbo implants. Nearly 10 percent choose double D.

—ALEX KUSCZYNSKI, *BEAUTY JUNKIES*[26]

Women attempted to inflate the size of their breasts long before breast augmentation surgeries became available. Beginning in the late 1890s, doctors began to inject substances like paraffin, beeswax, and vegetable oil into women's breasts to enhance size. Ivory and glass, among other materials, were used as some of the first experimental implant devices. Early attempts to increase breast size by transplanting fat from other parts of the body were widely attempted and entirely unsuccessful.[27] It would take years before these procedures approximated today's common boob job. The great-great-grand-mammary of today's modern implant wasn't even born until the early 1960s. Implant surgeries have been on the rise ever since, only temporarily losing their appeal in the early 1990s when the U.S. Congress imposed limits on the use of silicone implants because they were thought to be harmful to women. Saline implants, though, remained a popular alternative and are still in use today.

Surveys claim that four million women now have breast implants: 80 percent elective and 20 percent reconstructive.[28] Despite these statistics, it's hard to gauge actual numbers. Physicians performing such surgeries aren't subject to any reporting requirements, and many aren't affiliated with any official board. Accurate numbers might not mean too much to the average person. After all, who cares whether there are 3 or 6 million pairs of augmented breasts in a population of 150 million U.S. women? But many people do think numbers matter and that the

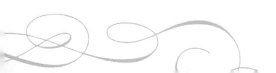

increased occurrence of larger boobs in our society sends the wrong message to girls and women. Some, like author Alex Kuczynski, are concerned that women who seek "porn-size" boobs represent the triumph of pornography in our society.[29]

According to surgeons, augmentation patients seem to fall into two categories: (1) small-breasted women in their twenties and thirties bothered by their lack of breast tissue, and (2) women aged thirty to fifty who, after childbearing or due to age, are unhappy with sagging and/or less-full-looking breasts. The average breast implant patient is often in her thirties, college educated, and married with children. Survey results show that 88 percent are happy with their results, and 93 percent would recommend the surgery to a friend or family member.[30] Studies also show that women with breast implants have lower risks of breast cancer, heart disease, and other major illnesses. But this group has also been found to have higher rates of suicide.[31] No one knows the exact reason why, but it's thought that higher rates of depression in some augmentation patients prior to surgery may be the root cause.[32]

"The typical augmentation patient I see chooses a large B or small C cup breast," says plastic surgeon Drew Welk of Seattle.[33] There is a growing trend toward breast augmentation, and such surgeries will probably increase with the recent FDA approval of a new generation of silicone implants. But no one can say whether those implants are of a medium size (to replace lost breast volume from pregnancy and age) or large (to supersize small to medium breasts). Even if one inflated breast augmentations to assume that ten million women now sport "fake" breasts, it still wouldn't account for the massive increase in naturally larger breasts, much of which may simply be due to a worldwide obesity epidemic. Surgeons do report, however, that many of their patients are concerned about drawing too much attention to themselves with breast implants and fear choosing too large a size. And yet, after their surgeries, nearly 40 percent wish they had gone "bigger."[34]

In the final analysis, breast surgeries seem to have more to do with how women see themselves than how they think society views their bodies. (Again, opponents of these procedures argue that a woman who believes she is making her breasts firmer and perkier for "herself" has merely internalized society's warped view of the female breast.[35]) The American Society of Plastic Surgeons admits to a rising trend among thirtysomething women, many of whom are undergoing "Mommy Makeovers," multiple surgeries after they've had children.[36] Since breasts are made of tissue and fat, augmentation may be the only option for some women determined to get back their pre-baby boobs.

MEN AND IMPLANTS: MIXED MESSAGES

Are men thrilled by the trend of women's breasts getting bigger? Some have taken the initiative and actively encouraged women to undergo breast augmentations. Consider the website My Free Implants, which assists women who can't afford augmentation surgeries. A woman can create an account and be paid $1 per message to chat with men who are sympathetic to her cause.[37] Theoretically, a woman can earn enough to pay for implants, the underlying message being that she'll

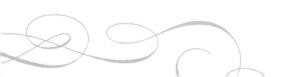

at least be willing to send her "benefactors" a thank-you photo of her new boobs. (In 2005, My Free Implants claims to have paid for seven augmentation procedures, although Alex Kuczynski only raised $96 over the course of three weeks when she created an account while researching her book.[38])

Despite this testosterone-driven show of generosity, *More* magazine in the U.K. ran a piece that stated that 85 percent of men think plastic surgery is a "complete turn-off." A spokeswoman for the magazine says, "Women would be better off spending their money on a new dress and shoes rather than fake breasts."[39] The American Society of Plastic Surgeons reports on the growing demand by thirty-something women for "Mommy Makeovers" (multiple cosmetic procedures such as liposuction, tummy tucks, and implants).[40] Even on such pro-augmentation sites as All About Breast Augmentation, surveys show that only 32 percent of U.S. men rate implants as a 10 on a scale of 1 to 10.[41]

Are men thrilled with the report trend of women seeking larger breasts?[42] In an article entitled "How Men Really Feel About Breast Implants," written for *O, The Oprah Magazine,* Tom Chiarella compares a woman with breast implants to a new car: "You can always feel the implant, and feeling it will always lead you to the conscious realization that someone pimped this breast."[43] The macho sentiment behind this comment might lead some women to roll their eyes. But there are other men out there who get that the choice is ultimately and more importantly about what the woman wants and not about what the male population wishes to see. Recalling his male friend's reaction to a partner's augmentation surgery, Chiarella acknowledged, "The implants solved something for her, not him."[44]

GENERAL BREAST EXPECTATIONS

I kept waiting for them to "bounce back" after nursing, refusing to believe they were gone—even though I never appreciated them. I call it restorative surgery. I'm now a cup bigger, still not comfortable with them ... but they look fabulous!
—34C/D (FORMERLY B), AGE 41

Your breasts are unique, and you and your surgeon must decide how best to meet your goals. As with any surgery, you need to weigh possible risks and complications against potential (but not guaranteed) results. Some procedures can result in excessive blood loss, infection, loss of nipple sensation (differs from woman to woman), and other problems specifically associated with implants. Check out the Boobliography in the appendix for books and other resources for greater guidance.

CHOOSING YOUR SURGEON

This will be your most important decision. Spend the time finding someone who listens to what you want, understands your perspective, and makes you feel comfortable. Keep in mind that you may have to return to her or him for future revisions. Interview several doctors and solicit recommendations from friends and other acquaintances. Do a background check on her or his medical credentials and make sure the doctor you choose has been certified by the American Board of Plastic Surgery (ABPS). (Anyone can be "board certified" by a legitimate-sounding organization, but only the ABPS holds the highest standards for certification.) Ask about privileges at a nearby hospital, in case of an emergency. During your consult, look at before and after photos of previous patients. You should feel free to ask questions and have them thoroughly answered. Ask if you can speak with former patients about their experiences.

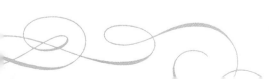

DECIDING ON A TIME AND PLACE

Whether you're going bigger, smaller, or getting a lift, your procedure will most likely be performed in the doctor's office, an outpatient surgical facility, or a hospital. Except in cases of breast reconstruction and some reductions, most cosmetic surgeries are performed on an outpatient basis, so you're back home the same day. General anesthesia is typically (but not always) used, and length of time to operate varies widely. One person's breast lift might take one to two hours, while another's could take five or six. Your doctor can give you a better estimate depending on your particular set of circumstances. (Keep in mind, speedy service doesn't necessarily correlate with best results.) You may also opt to have more than one procedure during the same operation, such as a breast lift with augmentation. Discuss the pros and cons of multiple surgeries with your doctor.

FIGURING OUT THE COST

With the exception of breast reconstruction, congenital deformities, and some—but not all—breast reductions, you will have to cover all surgical costs, including anesthesia and implant materials. These fees must be paid prior to surgery, although some practitioners offer credit plans. Most welcome the use of plastic (credit cards) to pay for plastic surgery. Rough estimates are listed in the following section by individual surgery and also vary widely.

DECIDING YOUR BREAST SIZE

If you're going bigger, or seeking reconstruction after an illness or accident, it's important to determine the best breast size and shape for your body. Both symmetry and proportion should be taken into consideration. A tall athletic woman might look fabulous with a D cup, but that same size may be out of place on a smaller-framed woman. Many women want their breasts placed close together, as a way to create "natural cleavage." But cleavage is not a naturally occurring state, and the only way to get it is by wearing a bra that shoves your boobs together. What you should aim for is as natural a look as possible in your everyday clothes (and not just the occasional plunging evening outfit).

Dr. Robert M. Freund, author of *Cosmetic Breast Surgery,* suggests breast augmentation patients use the "rice test." Fill two plastic bags with uncooked rice—squeezing out any excess air—and lay them against your breasts inside your bra. He then recommends that women try different amounts of rice over the course of a week and vary their clothing choices from sweaters to tight T-shirts. This may give you a better idea of what size feels comfortable to you. It also provides guidance to your surgeon on what you believe will fit you best.[45]

FACING CHANGING BREAST REALITIES

If you've decided to have your breasts reduced, artificially expanded, or propped up, it's important to know that they won't remain that way forever. Losing or gaining weight, getting pregnant, or just the good old laws of gravity all work against these thousand-dollar procedures. Women with large implants may decide they want them reduced, or removed, as they grow older. Breast reduction patients may gain a few pounds and find it's gone right to their boobs. Excessive scar tissue or implant problems might require a future operation. The best possible surgical result does not translate into your boobs remaining the same the rest of your life.

KNOW YOUR SURGERIES

Here's a list of the most common procedures women undergo, including what to expect, how much they cost, and some concerns associated with each surgery.[46] This is an overview, so if and when you decide to get serious about going through with any one of these procedures, do further research, starting with the recommendations listed in the Boobliography.

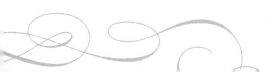

BREAST AUGMENTATION (AUGMENTATION MAMMOPLASTY)

This cosmetic procedure enhances small breasts, or creates fullness that may have been lost due to pregnancy, weight loss, or aging. Implants are made of a silicone shell filled with saline (saltwater) or silicone. Many women and doctors prefer silicone implants because they are thought to produce more "natural" results. However, no implant "feels" like a natural breast, and the degree to which it looks natural is more a matter of size and how it's placed.

When considering breast augmentation, you'll be asked to choose the following:

- type of implant, silicone or saline (and whether to "overfill" if you choose saline, as a means to reduce deflation)
- size and shape of implant
- location (placed over or under the muscle)
- implant texture (ribbed or smooth, although this isn't visible after surgery)
- incision location (around the nipple, under the arm, through the belly button, or under the breast)

Each of the above has its own pros and cons, depending on your particular situation. For instance, implant placement below the muscle can lend a better aesthetic result and interferes less with mammography imaging, but it may also be more painful and awkward. Make sure to get the boob scoop on all your options.

Approximate Cost
$4,000–$8,000

Common Concerns
- "Capsular contracture" refers to scar tissue that inevitably forms around the implant. If it's severe, it can cause the breast to feel

hard (due to scar tissue, not the implant). This condition can occur right after or years following surgery, and no one knows why it occurs in some women and not others.

- Ability to breastfeed may be reduced, depending on placement of implants and other factors.
- Connective tissue diseases such as lupus and rheumatoid arthritis were reported to be associated with silicone (but not saline) implants, which led to their removal from the U.S. market in the early 1990s. No scientific studies have ever found a link between silicone implants and such diseases.[47]

BREAST LIFT (MASTOPEXY)

This cosmetic procedure reshapes sagging breasts by removing skin but not breast tissue. The most common method involves a "key hole" incision where the surgeon cuts around the nipple, downward and underneath the breast. Loose skin is removed, and the areola is reduced in size and moved up onto the newly formed breast shape. A lift is often done in conjunction with breast augmentation to increase or restore breast size.

Approximate Cost

$5,000–$10,000

Common Concerns

- Scarring can be more prominent with a breast lift.
- Nipple sensitivity can be affected; it may be temporary or permanent.
- Additional sagging can lead to a "bottoming out" effect, making the nipple look too high on the breast.

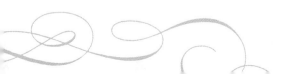

BREAST REDUCTION (REDUCTION MAMMOPLASTY)

Often covered through insurance, this surgery reduces the size of too-large or too-heavy breasts by removing actual breast tissue, not just loose skin. This may relieve a number of physical problems, such as back and neck pain. Different methods are used and many result in an "anchor" shaped scar similar to the one that results from a breast lift. Size, breast shape, and degree of sagging are all factors in determining what technique is best to reduce your breasts.

Approximate Cost

$6,000–$12,000 *(Check with your insurance company, since criteria used to determine eligibility for this procedure are not uniform. Some insurance carriers only cover the procedure if a specific amount of tissue is removed, regardless of the patient's height and weight.)*

Common Concerns

- Ability to breastfeed may be impacted, although 50 percent of breast reduction patients do go on to nurse.[48]
- Nipple sensitivity can be reduced, or lost completely, if the areola cannot simply be moved up on the breast but must be detached from existing tissue and grafted back in place.
- Scarring may be more obvious, depending on the type of incision.

BREAST RECONSTRUCTION

Even though insurance companies are now mandated by law to pay for breast reconstruction after a mastectomy, less than 20 percent of eligible women opt for the procedure. The older a women is when she receives a mastectomy, the less likely she is to undergo reconstruction. Less than half of these surgeries are performed on women age fifty and older.[49] Some women also prefer the ease of a breast prosthesis and see no need to undergo additional surgery. Others feel no need to even wear a bra and are satisfied to live their lives without breasts. For others, reconstruction can help in their own healing process and make them feel more "normal" after going through diagnosis and treatment for cancer.

For women who do choose reconstruction, timing can be an issue. Some doctors encourage women to have surgery at the same time as their mastectomy. Others believe it's more reasonable to wait. Dr. Drew Welk, a plastic surgeon specializing in cosmetic breast and reconstructive surgeries, believes that "a woman who just received a diagnosis of cancer may be overwhelmed both physically and emotionally and may not comprehend additional reconstruction information."[50] Complications may arise when combining one or more surgeries. Some women with a single mastectomy may have surgery to reshape the other healthy breast and thus match a rebuilt counterpart. While there are some skin-sparing mastectomies that allow women to retain some breast tissue, and possibly the nipple, in most of these surgical procedures all sensation in the breast and nipple area is lost.

There are two primary ways in which a woman can have reconstruction surgery after a mastectomy. The first is the "flap" method, which involves taking muscle and tissue from another part of the body (such as the back, abdomen, or buttocks) and transferring it to the chest wall. This method leads to more scarring on the body, simply due to the additional surgery. The other method involves the use of silicone or saline breast implants. First, a "tissue expander" is placed under the chest muscle and inflated over several weeks. The surgeon then places the implant under the muscle and fashions a nipple out of skin, which can then be tattooed to make the coloring more similar to the original nipple. Which procedure a woman is eligible for depends on her specific breast cancer treatment or whether she has enough additional body tissue to utilize the "flap" method.[51]

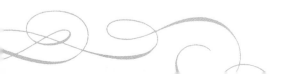

POTENTIAL SURGICAL ANSWERS TO
SPECIFIC BREAST CONCERNS

- **Inverted nipples.** Inverted nipples result from shortened milk ducts in the breast pulling the entire nipple "in." Surgery can be performed that pulls the tissue back out, but this will affect a woman's ability to breastfeed since milk ducts must be severed in the process.

- **Enlarged areolaes.** Some women are happy with the way their breasts look but don't like the size of their areolas, especially after they finish breastfeeding. This can be reduced by removing excess skin.

- **Severe breast asymmetry.** All women have asymmetrical breasts, but approximately 10 percent develop severe asymmetry during puberty.[52] These women's breasts may vary widely in size, with one much larger than the other, often by more than one 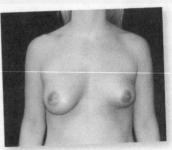 cup size. Sometimes the breasts are shaped differently. This can make girls self-conscious, not to mention the difficulties in finding well-fitting bras or swimwear. Plastic surgery can reduce one breast, or make the other an equal size by inserting an implant. Insurance companies don't all agree that such surgery is medically necessary, so you'll have to check with your individual insurance carrier to determine coverage for such an operation.

Dr. Lisa Lynn Sowder

- **Tubular or hypoplastic breasts.** This condition is thought to be caused by a scarcity of breast tissue and results in a woman's breasts being more tubular than round. Many

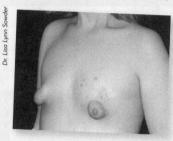

Dr. Lisa Lynn Sowder

women with tubular breasts are perfectly happy but experience problems breastfeeding. The lack of breast tissue makes it more difficult to produce milk. While plastic surgery is often recommended to change the look of tubular breasts (through lifts and implants), it does not improve the ability to nurse and could in fact make it more difficult. If you're considering surgery to correct this, you may want to wait until after you finish breastfeeding. Since it is classified as a medical condition, reconstructing tubular breasts could be covered under some medical plans.

- **Poland's syndrome.** This rare condition is evident at birth and occurs when breast tissue and even underlying muscles are missing from one side of a girl's body. Many women with Poland's syndrome will choose plastic surgery as a way to reconstruct the "missing" breast tissue. Surgery to correct such conditions found at birth is typically considered medically necessary. These surgeries are often performed on adolescents at the time when normal breast tissue is developing or complete.

TROUBLING TEEN TREND OR MEDIA HYPE?

20/20 reporter John Stossel looked into the camera and asked, "Why are parents buying their girls the gift of surgery?" and proceeded to recount the stories of countless teens who are receiving breast implants as high school graduation presents.[53] Websites such as Hilary.com condemn the trend of "Surgery as Sweet 16 Gift" and the rising number of girls under eighteen undergoing breast augmentation surgery with the approval of their parents.[54] Is this a trend worthy of public concern or just a case of the media making something of nothing?

The American Society of Plastic Surgeons reports that 329,386 breast augmentations were performed in 2006 in the United States. Teenagers under the age of nineteen accounted for 9,104 of those procedures (3 percent of the total—up 12 percent since 2005). By contrast, 13,900 young men under eighteen had breast reduction (gynecomastia) surgery in 2006, up 21 percent from 2005. Another 6,529 women under the age of nineteen also had breast reductions, out of a total of 104,455, in 2006.[55]

The American Academy of Cosmetic Surgery cautions parents about breast augmentation surgery for teen girls, advising that those wishing to do so for purely cosmetic reasons should wait until they are eighteen. They recommend that young women should be fully developed, both physically and emotionally.[56]

SILICONE WARS

Silicone was first used during World War II when Japanese prostitutes had it injected into their breasts in order to attract the attention of American soldiers.[57] These injections weren't always legal but became popular in the United States and helped boost the busts of topless dancers and some starlets through the early 1960s. Not everyone realized that liquid silicone could migrate to other parts of the body, in some cases resulting in infection and amputation of the breast.[58] Everyday women even submitted to risky shots from door-to-door salesmen posing as doctors.

Early versions of the silicone implant that were first used in 1962 were introduced before FDA approval was required for such medical devices.[59] They were touted as safe throughout the 1970s and '80s. And by the 1970s, mastectomy patients began using them for breast reconstructions. In the late 1980s and early 1990s, stories from women about high rates of capsular contracture, silicone bleed (when silicone leaks from the sac into the body), and links to autoimmune disease began to appear the media. In 1992, due in large part to these reports, the FDA restricted silicone implants to breast reconstruction patients. A successful class-action suit against Dow Corning, the largest implant manufacturer, forced the company into bankruptcy in 1995.[60] Since that time, a comprehensive study has shown there is no link between connective tissue diseases and silicone implants.[61] The fourteen-year-old implant ban was lifted by the FDA in November of 2006 when it approved the use of a new generation of implants. The FDA has warned that these implants are not risk-free, and women will need regular MRI screenings for the rest of their lives to monitor possible implant ruptures.[62]

LIVING WITH YOUR NEW BREAST SELF

I love their bigger size—C/D—and sometimes I hate it. It's like driving a Porsche full-time. Cool when you want to look cool, but out of place going to the grocery store. Sometimes I miss my "cute" size Bs for all those tiny summer tops, but I look fabulous in a sweater!

−34 C/D (FORMERLY B), AGE 41

Even women who've done a lot of research on what breast surgery entails may be surprised by how it feels to live life with now-unfamiliar breasts. Your new boobs may represent the first time in your life that you're breasts will be "big," "small," or "just right." And adjusting to

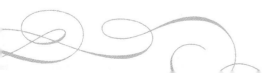

new breasts will continue for years to come. In the aftermath of breast surgery, it's good to liken it to a new adolescence, especially since these "new" breasts are as subject to change as the old ones.

GET TO KNOW YOUR NEW GIRLS

Post-op breasts will feel different to you and your lover's touch. Women with implants often have to readjust to such simple tasks as hugging a friend or rolling over in bed. You may not be able to pass a mirror without staring at your new silhouette in disbelief. It may take a while to register this new breast self as your normal appearance. You'll also have to get to know your girls again, on an ongoing basis. Changing scar tissue makes it difficult to determine what are now normal lumps and bumps in your breasts. Breast self-exams should be more important than ever, if only as a way to acquaint yourself with your new girls.

NEW SIZE, CHOICES, AND CHALLENGES

Clothing retailers in some warmer states, where breast augmentations are more popular, report an increased number of alterations to accommodate suddenly bigger-busted patients.[63] Those shaving off a cup size or two may find it easier to buy off the rack for their now smaller racks. But many women fail to factor in the cost of a new wardrobe when considering a change in their boob size. Some breast surgery patients may find they are less inhibited after their surgery and may reveal their breast selves to anyone who asks. If they never felt comfortable wearing low-cut tops prior to their procedure, increased cleavage may result in a greater willingness to show off their girls. Some women may find they are criticized for flaunting their surgically enhanced breasts.

bOOb*flash!*

**WARMER WEATHER STATES BRING OUT THE
BREAST IN COSMETIC PLASTIC SURGERY**

The American Society of Plastic Surgeons reports
that 36 percent of all augmentations in the United
States are performed in the region that includes
Arizona, California, Nevada, and Hawaii![64]

PARTNERS' REACTION TO NEW BREAST SELF

Time and time again, plastic surgeons report that partners—no matter whether they were initially opposed to plastic surgery—are overwhelmingly pleased with results. This may have everything to do with a woman's increased self-esteem and self-confidence. But some women complain about their partners' obvious enthusiasm for new boobs. They often resent their partners taking too much pleasure in something that was not done for their benefit.

DUE BOOB-DILIGENCE

Surgery to change breasts is sometimes called "cosmetic," implying it's as easy and simple as putting on makeup. But it is serious and irreversible and will forever change how your breasts look and feel. If you choose implants, you must accept their inevitable higher maintenance and potential future complications and/or replacement. Just like face lifts, or noncosmetic surgeries such as knee replacements, nothing lasts a lifetime. You should have reasonable expectations about outcomes, because there is no "ideal breast" except your own.

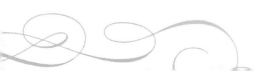

CHAPTER TWELVE

The More Mature Breast: Saggy, Yet Sexy & Sassy

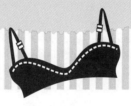

I am what I am—not too bad for a middle-aged gal.
—34B, AGE 48

They've somehow made it through pregnancy, nursing, and weight fluctuations in decent shape. Not the perkiest, but they've held up pretty well. What seemed impossibly pendulous on a sixteen-year-old girl seems almost perky on a forty-two-year-old woman.
—36C, AGE 42

WELCOME TO THE OLDER BOOB GENERATION

The world's population is getting older, due both to a decline in fertility and an increase in average life span. The number of people over sixty-five is predicted to increase from 12 percent in 2000 to nearly 20 percent in 2030.[1] Our older breasts may have plenty of company, but experts also believe that our longevity will put a real strain on health and other long-term care. It may be challenging for the medical infrastructure to meet the growing demands of mammography screening (if that continues to be the best detection method available for the next quarter century). Perhaps we'll see this demographic shift result in a booming market of bras targeted to elderly women.

According to a 2005 AARP study, the majority of women over forty-five are happier than they have ever been. They look at aging as a great way to pursue new dreams and do things they've always wanted to do. Most speak of having at least one older role model who they look to as a source of inspiration.[2] The wisdom of age does lead to greater self-awareness and self-confidence. And aging boob owners have other advantages over the younger breast generation. After menopause, women are less likely to suffer from depression—just another indication that getting past our reproductive years may offer some women a newfound sense of stability.[3]

Considering how far removed the older breast is from our society's young and perky ideal, it may come as a surprise to learn that plenty of women are perfectly happy with their more mature bosoms. Many are pleased with where theirs land in middle age, whether they've changed or not with pregnancy, breastfeeding, or through alterations like plastic surgery. Women who have faced breast cancer, or have a relative or friend dealing with the disease, will likely view their lives and their breasts in a different light. Since age is one of the greatest risk factors for breast cancer, older women become more accustomed to helping others through illnesses related to breasts. And these are the types of experiences that make us more accepting of the journey our boobs continue to go through as we age.

We know that our worth does not rest in the size or shape of our chests. Our breasts are more interesting because they are not viewed solely as sexual objects (although some of us do like to show them off on occasion). They've blended into the rest of our bodies and our lives. The biggest challenge we face, given the softer look of our breasts, is trying to find a bra that makes them look good in our clothes. But we're also more patient with our girls than we used to be, and we've learned to accept these challenges in our own way. We know our breasts have served us in many different ways during the course of our lives and thank them for coming along for the ride.

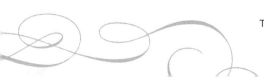

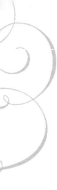

MORPHING MOUNDS THROUGH MENOPAUSE

Because of the hormonal changes associated with perimenopause, many
women experience breast pain, especially during the second half of the
menstrual cycle . . . often breast pain comes and goes seemingly at random.

—Christiane Northrup[5]

Menopause can feel a lot like puberty, except backward. This time around, instead of being constantly concerned about what others think about your development, you might feel the exact opposite. Only your opinion counts. By the time we reach our fifties, we've experienced enough biological fluctuations to accept a few more. And many of us may look forward to an end to the roller-coaster ride that's marked our reproductive years, even though many of us have to endure years of living through "the change."

Menopause can cause raging hormonal shifts, and some women go through periods of breast swelling and painful lumpiness. Angie, a fifty-seven-year-old 38DD, commented that she felt like she "could bake a loaf of bread under each breast" during her flashes. "They have finally calmed a bit, but I can still count on at least three 'heat' episodes a night." Night sweats, insomnia, and other discomforts during menopause can cause some women to seek relief through hormone replacement or bioidentical hormones. But some of these drugs, in certain doses, have been linked to higher rates of breast cancer (see sidebar, The Great Hormone Replacement Therapy Debate). It might be worth it to try herbal remedies, which some women do find helpful. For others, there may be no relief from irritating symptoms; they may have to tough out this phase of their life (not unlike puberty) until this final fluctuating boob phase ends.

"As women get older, the breasts tend to sag and flatten; the larger the breasts, the more they sag. For some women, however, menopause can bring with it an enormous increase in the size of their breasts," says Dr. Miriam Stoppard in *Breast Health*.[6] In our postmeno-pausal years, glandular, dense breast tissue is replaced by fatty tissue. For some women, that could mean an increase in breast size, while it's the opposite for others. It all depends on how much and where fat comes to rest in an individual woman's breasts. The good news is that if your breasts become less dense, it may be easier to find irregularities through mammography. Detecting such signs of breast cancer sooner, as mentioned in Chapter 10: In Sickness and in Health, is one of the primary factors in increased survival rates. Gravity may take its toll on where our breasts rest, but there are other advantages for which we can be thankful.

TITS OF WISDOM

My breasts are fine. I'm fairly heavy, which means my breasts are large and would probably be the first thing to go were I to lose weight. I feel very attached to my breasts.
—36C, AGE 52

Here's the good news about older breasts: Most women feel far more comfortable carrying them on their aging bodies. If we haven't adapted or adjusted to their nature and are still uncomfortable, we now have the maturity to deal with the situation. Sally, a sixty-eight-year-old D cup, recalls: "For years I talked about getting a breast reduction. Of course, all of my husbands—I've had three; once divorced, twice widowed—said, 'No way, I love them.' I suggested they might want to carry them around! I always wanted to lose weight before I had anything done, and now that I am more determined, perhaps I will consider the surgery more seriously." Lots of older women are paying for the pair they wished they'd had their entire lives. Whether the procedure involves a lift, implants, or a reduction, women are choosing to change their breasts to please themselves. One

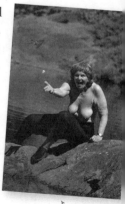

Jordan Matter

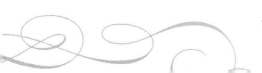

fifty-year-old woman was delighted with her results and said, "They are no longer saggy and uneven. The modern miracles of plastic surgery have overcome what nature gave me."

Other women find that having the perspective of age has caused them to look at their own breasts differently, and that in itself provides a great lift. Jackie, who's forty-six and very well endowed, relates that aging hasn't made that much of a difference. "They were never cute and perky to begin with, so there's no change of body image to deal with." Another sixty-one-year-old provides an honest and forthright point of view: "My breasts certainly do not stand up the way they did when I was young, but they are still sexy, and I enjoy having them." Teri, a DD who just turned fifty, says, "I wouldn't mind having them lifted, but I actually like them because they balance out the ravages of age on the lower half of my body." Many larger women simply appreciate their breasts for what they are. "They're my favorite part of my body," declares Monique, a forty-six-year-old 34D. Kathy, who's sixty-one and a DD, says, "I think my breasts are great. They are very sexy, and I love the way they flow." A fifty-year-old D cup, whose mother had two mastectomies, now sees her breasts through another set of eyes: "My breasts are fine—quite saggy, cancer-free so far, and my husband loves them." Many women are able to let go of self-criticism as they age. Getting older allows us to be focused on more-important things, like being happy to have breasts that have made it this far.

SISTERS SLUMP

Some breasts get saggy sooner. There's nothing wrong with this scenario, and it may have more to do with inherited skin elasticity than with gravity's power to send our girls farther south.

While older small-breasted women may have wished that they were a slightly bigger size at some point in their lives, many are happy with how their breasts have fared over time. "I'm not big enough to be saggy, so they are as good as new. I appreciate being flat and buy bras with padding so I can fill out my clothes," says one forty-seven-year-old B cup. "I'm perky as ever," says a fifty-six-year-old whose petite size allows her to comfortably not wear bras. A fifty-one-year-old A cup echoes a similarly chirpy sentiment: "They still look great, small and high on my chest." A slightly bigger fifty-five-year-old B cup sums it up this way: "They are firm, sexy, and sassy. I feel I owe it all to going braless." Whether it's genetics, skin elasticity, size, or simply choosing to not wear a bra, all of these women feel good about their breasts at a later stage of life.

BEHOLD THE WONDERS OF THE RIGHT BRA

I'm built low, which wasn't a problem into my thirties, but now that I'm in my late fifties, gravity has really lowered my profile. I find it difficult to find a bra that puts my breasts up enough to keep me from looking like someone from the 1880s.

—42C, AGE 57

With greater age, comes greater acceptance of what we think are the best breasts possible, be they saggy, full, flat, or still somewhat perky. They are tied less to society's views of what constitutes the best size and shape of breasts. Most women have no desire to turn the clock back or to trade a high-riding set for the ones that have been with them through thick and thin, or in sickness and in health. (Although it's true that some women who got larger implants at an earlier age tend to dial theirs down to a smaller size as they grow older.) But no matter how far we've come in accepting the breasts we have, no one underestimates their value as a fashion accessory.

Getting the right bra fit for your girls is part of helping them look their very best in your clothes. Many women find that their boob flesh and placement changes with age. What used to rest higher and in front may seem to gravitate sideways, resting closer to the armpits. Victoria Roberts of Zovo Lingerie advises that, at a certain point, it's no longer about pushing our boobs together to create great cleavage. "Older women will get beautiful décolletage if they choose a bra that lifts and separates. The last thing you want to do is place them side by side, all crunched together, creating a monoboob look." In her experience, those with greater horizontal breast tissue do well with a demicup bra. While this bra is often recommended for younger women, it also works for softer, pliable skin by holding

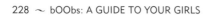

SuzyLamont.com

TONE AND FIRM FOR BETTER BREAST HEALTH

Exercise is the best way to prolong your life and keep your body feeling and looking younger. And it's never too late to get started on the road to fitness. Studies show that older women who do strength training see great improvement when it comes to building stronger bones and losing weight.[10] Exercise also improves muscle mass and contributes to better balance in postmenopausal women.[11]

Most important for our breast health is the fact that simple weight training can do wonders for building proper posture and toning arms and backs, all of which complement our breasts. Many older women find that it's easier to exercise with a bosom buddy, so think about joining up with a friend to start in a program of firming and toning to benefit your overall health.

the breast tissue in each cup without pressing them tightly together. Many demicup bras (sometimes also called balconnet bras) come in beautiful lace patterns, which can add a touch of sensuality to the more mature woman's wardrobe. If you don't like the look of lace showing through your blouse, consider purchasing some silky camisoles to smooth out your silhouette.

Another challenge for less-full breasts are those molded cup bras that might have fit nicely premenopause but leave too much room at the top of the bra cup afterward. Going down one cup size may be all the change you need to get your girls comfortable again. Because the band is where you get all your support, some elderly gals think they should wear a larger band to prevent pressure on their skin and the appearance of back fat through clothing. But having this area snug will keep your girls from slouching, so consider buying some thin underpinnings if you want to smooth out your look. Whatever you do, make sure you spend some time with a professional fitter to

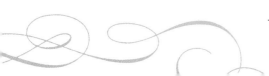

determine the best kind of bra for you at this stage in your life. As your breasts change, so do their needs. Don't think that the bra that best fit you a year ago is going to be right for you now. Find a lingerie store that caters to the more mature boob owner. You may have to spend a bit more on lingerie, but it's worth it when you're paying for comfort. The good news is that when you're past menopause (and any hormonal supplements), you won't have to worry as much about monthly size fluctuations.

HONORING THE MORE MATURE BREAST

It would be nice to have the perfect young breasts again, but I'm more concerned about their health than sex appeal.

−34C, AGE 52

After fifty-plus years of dealing with her own breasts, Lydia, age seventy, concludes that what makes her happiest is knowing that her breasts are healthy. She doesn't mind the yearly poking and prodding at the doctor's or the annual squashing mammogram because of the peace of mind it gives her to know that if a problem arises, she can deal with it right away. Keeping on top of yearly exams is one of the best ways to honor your more mature breasts. You also want to watch for the onset of any of the benign breast conditions, described in Chapter 10: In Sickness and in Health. Older women with silicone breast implants should undergo regular MRI screenings to ensure that they stay intact. In addition to incorporating detection into your normal routine, you should focus on prevention. Everything you do to better your physical self, such as eating a balanced diet and getting regular exercise, will contribute to a longer and healthier life. By focusing on what's best for your whole body, you're contributing to better breast health as well.

Dragging your girls to the doctor's office once a year isn't the only way to show them some love. If you've had mixed feeling about your breasts in the past, now is a good time to make amends with your mammaries. Take the time to pamper them with lotion or a nice skin massage. They belong to you and are yours to enjoy as you wish. If you need some inspiration on how other postmenopausal women take pride in their breasts, explore some of the videos, calendars, and books recommended in the Boobliography. Some of these feature amazing women who pay tribute to the body and breast as beautiful at any size, shape, or age.

A breast that has stood the test of time deserves to be celebrated. Your girls may be older, but they're certainly more refined, too. For many of us, aging may mean that our breasts finally fit with the rest of our bodies. Some of us may have felt that we were born with more-mature-looking breasts and have now physically grown into them. As we grow older, our breasts are no longer viewed by others as the focal point of our sexuality (even though they still provide sexual pleasure), which can be a relief for some and hard to swallow for others. Our girls may have served in several capacities over the course of our lives, succeeding in some areas more than others. All that remains is our own breast flesh, which we can admire for its resilience and tenacity. They've hung in there through thick and thin, and they deserve a hearty round of applause.

Confessions of a Boobatologist

Let me get something off my chest. This book has had its ups and downs, not unlike my own breasts. It hasn't been easy, either, taking a budding idea and morphing it into a bigger platform. But there were always things that pumped me up: talking with teens about bra sizing, having total strangers tell me their own breast stories, and what I discovered through my research: that women's breasts are a fascinating and complex subject.

The more I researched, the more I was forced to toss out my own preconceived notions about breasts—like a ratty old bra. For instance, why are boobs growing bigger worldwide? Statistics on breast augmentations were too low to account for the difference. But bra manufacturers have introduced more buxom lines to meet demand. The only evidence supporting the idea that women's breasts are getting bigger are studies that show women, in general, have grown larger. No surprise that these gains are seen in a place that's more prone to storing fat deposits.

Visits to lingerie stores were a highlight of my work. Bras have confused and confounded me all my life: wires popping out of seams, bra straps cutting into shoulders, bands stretching out of place. Now I know that those problems have more to do with the way I cared for my lingerie than with a poorly fitted brassiere. My teenage daughter has benefited from my new expertise, since I don't hesitate to buy her more-expensive, well-made foundations.

Since my mother's premenopausal bout with breast cancer puts me at higher risk, I've been getting yearly mammograms since age

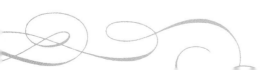

thirty, but I discovered that 80 percent of all breast cancer diagnoses are in women with no family history of the disease. I am more likely to die of heart disease than breast cancer.

Men's attitudes about breasts were yet another eye-opener. I still harbor memories of boys and men making uncouth comments about the larger breasts of my youth. When I asked male friends to weigh in on the subject, many stared back at me boob-struck. They were more comfortable looking at breasts than discussing them (at least with a woman, anyway). But many answered my questions and confirmed what others before me had found: Men love breasts. Maybe it has nothing to do with some fanciful theory of evolution. Maybe it is, as one adorable seventh-grade boy told me, "Because they are beautiful." I believe he's right.

I've discovered that every woman must decide what is "normal" for her own breasts. You can't appreciate the inherent beauty or magical qualities of your breasts if you accept only a narrow definition of their purpose. After all, one woman may choose to wear a bra; another may not. Some enjoy the experience of breastfeeding; others find it impossible. Still others may elect to have plastic surgery as a way to correct their relationship to their breasts, while some choose to have their breasts removed so they can be less concerned with their future health. There is no right or wrong way to live with breasts, just a continuously changing path—and it's a journey that's only enjoyable if we embrace their evolving, amazing nature.

This guide to your girls turned out every bit as unique as my own set. It started out small, smooth, and perky and grew bigger, grander, and bumpier. Adding more chapters rounded things out, but I had to deal with occasional sagginess. Other women's stories supported and uplifted the work. Our collective boobs are a true testament to how we meet the challenges of our lives. Breasts are gorgeous, powerful, nurturing, life-sustaining, sexy, funny, and ever-changing. Boobs rock. And the women attached to them? Even more.

Your Boob IQ Score

Add up the points for each of your answers and read your score below!

1.	a-1	b-0	c-2
2.	a-1	b-2	c-0
3.	a-0	b-2	c-1
4.	a-2	b-1	c-0
5.	a-2	b-1	c-0
6.	a-2	b-1	c-0
7.	a-1	b-2	c-0
8.	a-1	b-0	c-2
9.	a-0	b-1	c-2
10.	a-0	b-1	c-2
11.	a-2	b-1	c-0
12.	a-2	b-1	c-0
13.	a-1	b-0	c-2
14.	a-1	b-0	c-2
15.	a-2	b-1	c-0
16.	a-1	b-0	c-2
17.	a-1	b-2	c-0
18.	a-2	b-1	c-0

15 POINTS OR MORE: IGNORANCE IS NOT BLISS

You're probably wearing the wrong-size bra, or you've never been professionally fitted. It's not like you don't care; it's just that you've got other priorities in life. Look at it this way: You wouldn't wear uncomfortable shoes without making some adjustments, so give your

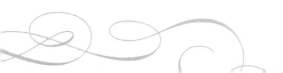

girls a break! Start now. The right bra isn't the only way to feel better about your very breast self. Learn what experts say you need to do to keep them happy and healthy throughout your life.

5–15 POINTS: WARMING UP TO YOUR GIRLS

You think your breasts are good, but not great. They don't get in your way, and some days you're thrilled to be their proud owner. But you have a few nagging questions. Maybe there are things you'd like to know so you'll be prepared for them in the future. Your inquisitive, positive, open attitude makes you ready to put your best breast forward in life.

0–5 POINTS: HIP TO YOUR TITS

Congratulations! You are in love with your ladies. You take care of them, and they take care of you. A girl like you keeps up with the latest boob news, so your pair is getting the best support possible. Keep up the great work!

Your Personal Boob Journal

Welcome to your personal boob journal. Here you can keep track of bra purchases, fittings, and breast exams and even map the topography of your own breasts. If you run out of room, simply download additional blank pages at www.booksonboobs.com. Congratulations on being good to your girls!

BRA RECORD

Keeping a record of when you bought a bra—or your last fitting—will help you determine when you need to replenish your boob wardrobe. Feel free to create your own rating system so you can reorder those that are the most beloved of the bunch.

Date	Size	FittingY/N	Style/Color/Manufacturer	Rating (*****)

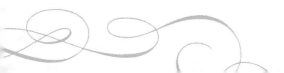

BREAST ASSESSMENTS

Record your breast self-exams, clinical breast exams, yearly mammogram, and breast MRIs below.

Doctor name/Phone number:

Date	BSE	CBE	Mammogram	MRI	Comments

Doctor name/Phone number:

Date	BSE	CBE	Mammogram	MRI	Comments

Doctor name/Phone number:

Date	BSE	CBE	Mammogram	MRI	Comments

Doctor name/Phone number:

Date	BSE	CBE	Mammogram	MRI	Comments

HOW TO DO A BREAST SELF-EXAMINATION (BSE)

In the Shower
Fingers flat, move gently over every part of each breast. Use your right hand to examine your left breast, left hand for right breast.

Check for any lump, hard knot, or thickening. Carefully observe any changes in your breasts.

Before a Mirror
Inspect your breasts with arms at your sides. Next, raise your arms high overhead.

Look for any changes in contour of each breast, a swelling, a dimpling of skin, or changes in the nipple. Then rest palms on hips and press firmly to flex your chest muscles. Left and right breasts will not exactly match—few women's breasts do.

Lying Down
Place pillow under right shoulder, right arm behind your head. With fingers of left hand flat, press right breast gently in small circular motions, moving vertically or in a circular pattern covering the entire breast. Use light, medium, and firm pressure. Squeeze nipple; check for discharge and lumps. Repeat these steps for your left breast.

MAP YOUR MAMMARIES
Keep track of the hills and valleys of your own girls using the diagrams on the next two pages. Mark any spots you find during your monthly breast self-exam, or fill it out with your healthcare provider during your annual clinical breast exam. Don't forget to include the date you mapped your mammaries!

BSE courtesy of the National Breast Cancer Foundation.

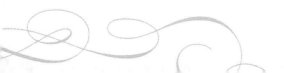

BOOB LOG, *Left Breast*

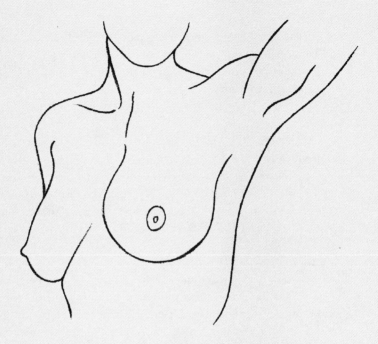

Tabitha Lahr

BOOB LOG, *Right Breast*

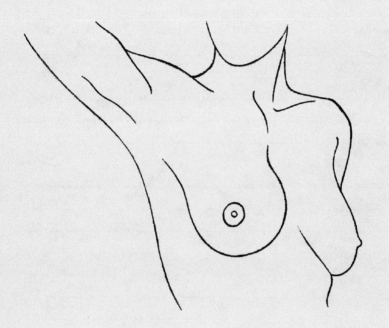

PERSONAL MAMMOIRS

Got something you'd like to get off your chest about your breasts? Use this page to jot down what amuses or confuses you about your boobs. Feel free to include drawings of your own bosom buddies!

_____

_____

_____

_____

_____

_____

_____

_____

_____

_____

_____

_____

_____

_____

_____

_____

_____

_____

_____

_____

_____

_____

All the Breast Resources

Below are books and websites you may find useful as further breast resources. More information, including recommended boob-related blogs, can be found on the Resources page of my website at www.books onboobs.com. If you can't find what you're looking for, or have your own recommendations, please email me at mammoirs@gmail.com.

BREAST PERSPECTIVES
Books

Bodies and Souls: The Century Project, photography by Frank Cordelle (Heureka Productions, 2006). A nude photographic journey of women's bodies from birth to age ninety-four. Not about breasts, but a celebration of the true beauty in every woman, no matter her age, shape, or size.

The Breast Book: A Curious and Intimate History, by Lithe Sebesta and Maura Spiegel (Workman Publishing Co., 2002). Fun, funny little breast book with great trivia and historical facts about breasts.

Breasts: Our Most Public Private Parts, by Meema Spadola (Wildcat Canyon Press, 1998). Based on the author's video documentary below.

Breasts: The Women's Perspective on an American Obsession, by Carolyn Latteier (Harrington Park Press, 1998). Men and women discuss how breasts are viewed in our society.

Breasts: Women Speak About Their Breasts and Their Lives, by Daphna Ayalah and Isaac J. Weinstock (Summit Books, 1979). Black-and-white photos of breasts, accompanied by interviews with women pictured.

The Descent of Woman: The Classic Study of Evolution, by Elaine Morgan (Souvenir Press, 1985). Another perspective on how and why women's bodies evolved as they did.

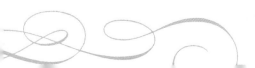

A History of the Breast, by Marilyn Yalom (Ballentine Books, 1997). A look at breasts through history, art, literature, and politics.

Master Breasts: Objectified, Aestheticized, Fantasized, Eroticized, Feminized by Photography's Most Titillating Masters..., by Francine Prose, Karen Finley, Dario Fo, and Charles Simic (Aperture Foundation, 1998). Breast photos from art and advertising like you've never seen before.

Woman: An Intimate Geography, by Natalie Angier (Anchor Books, 2000). A beautifully written and informative book from a Pulitzer Prize-winning author who does justice to the evolution of the female form. Her chapter on the story of the breast is titled "Circular Reasonings."

Videos and DVDs

Boobalogues: Our Breasts, Our Lives, by Kathy Kiefer (JACOL Filmworks, 2004). Documentary that covers the topics of breast development, breastfeeding, surgery, and cancer (www.boobalogues.com).

Breasts: A Documentary, HBO 1996, by Meema Spadola. A cinematic collection of "mammoirs," featuring interviews with twenty-two top-free boob owners from ages six to eighty-four. Includes stories from mothers/daughters, transsexuals, and mastectomy patients.

Busting Out, by Francine Strickwerda and Laurel Spellman Smith (Stir It Up Productions, 2004). Explores our society's fascination with breasts (www.bullfrogfilms.com).

Websites

007 Breasts
Breasts from every perspective, with information on breastfeeding and breast health, featuring a gallery of natural breast photos.
www.007b.com

American Association for Nude Recreation
Resource for information about nudist groups.
www.aanr.com

Cyber Angels
Organization dedicated to keeping kids safe on the Internet.
www.cyberangels.org

Feminist Majority Foundation
Resource on sexual harassment, including definitions and national hotlines.
www.feminist.org/911/harass.html

Naturist Action Committee
Nonprofit advocacy arm of the Naturist Society, working to protect the rights of naturists in North America.
www.nac.oshkosh.net

Topfree!
Provides information on where you can go top-free in the U.S. and around the world.
www.topfreedom.com

The Topfree Equal Rights Association (TERA)
Uncovers legal issues and efforts by women who wish to go top-free in the same manner men are allowed to be topless in public places in Canada and the United States.
www.tera.ca

This Is Beautiful
Gallery of beautiful nude photos of extraordinary women.
www.amandakoster.com/thisisbeautiful.org

Trade Association for Nude Recreation
Resource for clothing-optional destinations and organizations.
www.tanr.com/default.php?25

Uncovered: Busting Out in the Big Apple
Collection of photographs featuring bare-breasted women in public around New York City.
http://www.jordanmatter.com/

U.S. Equal Employment Opportunity Commission
Resource on workplace sexual harassment and how to report abuse.
www.eeoc.gov/types/sexual_harassment.html

Working to Halt Online Abuse (WHO@)
Volunteer organization helping to stop online abuse, includes both an adult and kid website.
www.haltabusektd.org (for kids and teens)
www.haltabuse.org (for adults)

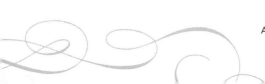

Books

101 Essential Tips: Breast Care, by Miriam Stoppard (DK Publishing, 1997). Small but very informative book on boobs that covers everything from breast health to bras and breast cancer.

Breast Fitness: An Optimal Exercise and Health Plan for Reducing Your Risk of Breast Cancer, by Anne McTiernan, MD, PhD; Julie Gralow, MD; and Lisa Talbott (St. Martin's Press, 2000). How to reduce your breast cancer risk through exercise, with detailed information on nutrition and lifestyle choices.

Breast Health, by Miriam Stoppard (DK Publishing, 1998). Compact resource filled with information on breast health.

Busting Out: Putting Your Best Breasts Forward, by Shirley Archer (Chronicle Books, 2007). Cute little book filled with exercises and "titbits" on how to keep your breasts in the best shape ever.

The Care & Keeping of You: The Body Book for Girls (American Girl Library), by Valorie Lee Schaefer (Pleasant Company Publications, 1998). Provides young girls (ages eight-twelve) with basics on how to take care of their growing bodies.

Changing Bodies, Changing Lives: A Book for Teens on Sex and Relationships, by Ruth Bell (Three Rivers Press, 1988). From the same folks who brought us *Our Bodies, Ourselves,* this is a great resource for older teens.

Deal With It! A Whole New Approach to Your Body, Brain, and Life as a gURL, by Esther Drill, Heather McDonald, and Rebecca Odes (Pocket Books, 1999). Great mature teen book from the creators of the gURL website. Includes information on breasts, bras, self-image, and creating your own personal style.

Dr. Susan Love's Breast Book, 4th ed., by Susan M. Love, MD, with Karen Lindsey (De Capo Press, 2005). *The New York Times* calls this the "bible" of breast books. This is a terrific medical resource and was recently revised and updated.

Our Bodies, Ourselves, by The Boston Women's Health Book Collective (Touchstone, 2005). Informative and enlightening discussions about general health issues, including body image and basic breast care.

Strength Training for Women, by Joan Pagano (DK Publishing, 2005). Illustrated guide on how to tone and firm muscles, with great upper-body exercises.

Weight Training for Dummies, by Liz Neporent, Suzanne Schlosberg, and Shirley Archer (Wiley Publishing, 2006). Comprehensive how-to guide on weight training, including building upper-body muscles.

What's Happening to My Body? Book for Girls: A Growing Up Guide for Parents and Daughters, by Lynda Madaras with Area Madaras (Newmarket Press, 2000). Includes personal stories and great illustrations for preteen and teen girls.

The Wisdom of Menopause: Creating Physical and Emotional Health During the Change, by Christiane Northrup, MD (Bantam, 2006). Covers topics of the aging breast, hormone therapy, and breast cancer prevention.

Websites

Breast of Canada
Information on breast health through a beautifully photographed calendar celebrating the diversity of women's breasts.
www.breastofcanada.com

Breast Self-Exam Video from Imaginis and Lange Productions
How to perform a monthly breast self-exam.
www.imaginis.com/breasthealth/bse_video.asp

Breast Self-Exam Video from Susan G. Komen for the Cure
Helpful BSE exam video in English and Spanish.
http://cms.komen.org/bse

The Breast Views
Daily news, education, and alternative views of the wonderful world of breasts, brought to you by Sue Richards, founder of Breast of Canada (see above).
http://thebreastviews.blogspot.com

The Breast Site
Features breast health products, services, and information.
www.thebreastsite.com

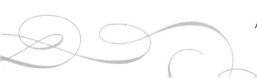

Breast Watch: The Boob FAQ
Great young-girl's guide to breasts and breast cancer, sponsored by Breast Cancer Watch.
http://boobwatch.evidencewatch.com

Check Your Boobies
Sign up here for a free monthly email reminder to check your boobies.
www.checkyourboobies.org

Imaginis
Resource for all breast-health-related topics, including benign breast disease.
www.imaginis.com

Woman's Touch MammoPad®
If pain or discomfort is holding you back from getting a mammogram, check out this helpful product.
www.biolucent.com/mammo.html

BREAST CANCER AND SUPPORT
Books

100 Questions & Answers About Breast Cancer, by Zora Brown and LaSalle D. Leffall Jr., MD, with Elizabeth Platt (Jones & Bartlett, 2003). Well-organized book covering questions regarding breast cancer.

Bathsheba's Breast: Women, Cancer & History, by James S. Olson (The John Hopkins University Press, 2002). History of breast cancer detection and treatment.

B.O.O.B.S.: A Bunch of Outrageous Breast Cancer Survivors Tell Their Stories of Courage, Hope and Healing, by Ann Kempner Fisher (Cumberland House, 2004). Stories from ten different breast cancer survivors.

Breast Cancer for Dummies, by Ronit Elk, PhD, and Monica Morrow, MD (Wiley Publishing, 2003). Practical and readable book about breast cancer.

Breast Cancer Husband: How to Help Your Wife (and Yourself) Though Diagnosis, Treatment and Beyond, by Marc Silver (Rodale Books, 2004). A manual on managing a breast cancer diagnosis as a couple, with dos and don'ts for men.

The Breast Cancer Survival Manual: A Step-by-Step Guide for the Woman with Newly Diagnosed Breast Cancer, 4th ed., by John Link, MD; Carey Cullinan, MD, MPH; Jane Kakkis, MD, MPH; and James Waisman, MD (Owl Books, 2007). Comprehensive guide on cancer definitions, genetic testing, and the importance of getting a second opinion.

The Breast Cancer Survivor's Fitness Plan, by Carolyn M. Kaelin, MD, MPH; Francesca Coltrera; Josie Gardiner; and Joy Prouty (McGraw-Hill, 2007). Includes fitness plan, exercises, and how to deal with lymphedema, lumpectomy, mastectomy, and breast reconstruction.

The Breast Cancer Wars: Hope, Fear, and the Pursuit of a Cure in Twentieth-Century America, by Barron H. Lerner, MD (Oxford Press, 2001). A history of the struggle to find a cure for breast cancer, highlighting how medical professionals and activists changed the way we approach breast cancer today.

Cancer Vixen: A True Story, by Marisa Acocella Marchetto (Knopf, 2006). A funny and moving graphic novel about breast cancer.

Just Get Me Through This! A Practical Guide to Coping with Breast Cancer, by Deborah A. Cohen and Robert M. Gelfand, MD (Kensington Books, 2000). Resource for women who have been diagnosed with early-stage breast cancer.

My One-Night Stand with Cancer, by Tania Katan (Alyson Books, 2005). Young gay woman's hilarious, enlightening, and inspiring memoir about her battle with breast cancer at twenty-one and thirty-one years of age.

Pink Ribbons, Inc.: Breast Cancer and the Politics of Philanthropy, by Samantha King (University of Minnesota, 2006). How pink ribbons became associated with breast cancer charities and the history and impact of cause-related marketing.

Uplift: Secrets from the Sisterhood of Breast Cancer Survivors, by Barbara Delinsky (Washington Square Press, 2003). Collection of stories from breast cancer survivors, including women's own survival secrets.

Whole: Women Healing Ourselves with Loving Energy, 12 Principles for Rebuilding Life after Breast Cancer, by Jacci Thompson-Dodd, MA, MSSS (Conch

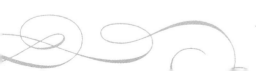

Shell Press, 2007). A book especially designed for African American women who have gone through breast cancer, but useful to anyone who has faced this disease.

Why I Wore Lipstick to My Mastectomy, by Geralyn Lucas (St. Martin's Griffin, 2005). Empowering and funny memoir of one young woman's battle with breast cancer. You can also download the movie based on the book at www.whyiworelipstick.com.

Websites

American Cancer Society
Information and resources on breast cancer, including clinical trials.
www.cancer.org

Avon Walk for Breast Cancer
Information on the three-day walk benefiting breast cancer.
http://walk.avonfoundation.org/

Breastcancer.org
Offers helpful and extensive discussion boards on specific issues related to breast cancer.
www.breastcancer.org

Breast Cancer Fund
Working to prevent and identify environmental causes of breast cancer.
www.breastcancerfund.org

Breast Cancer Watch
Provides the latest in evidence-based guidance on breast cancer therapies.
http://breastcancer.evidencewatch.com

Circus of Cancer
Inspiring site with practical information on how to help friends diagnosed with breast cancer.
www.circusofcancer.org

Imaginis
Information on breast cancer clinical trials.
www.imaginis.com/breasthealth/

Living Beyond Breast Cancer
> *A non-profit organization helping women with breast cancer. Includes information on clinical trials, message boards, and the latest news in breast cancer research.* www.lbbc.org.

National Breast Cancer Foundation, Inc.
> *Provides educational programs and funding for free mammograms for women who cannot afford them. Includes a resource library, group discussions, and form to help you build a support network in your own area.* www.nationalbreastcancer.org

National Lymphedema Network.
> *Provides education and guidance to lymphedema patients.* www.lymphnet.org

Susan G. Komen for the Cure
> *Dedicated to curing breast cancer, the organization provides resources on detection and treatment and holds numerous walks and runs to raise money for its foundation.* www.komen.org

Susan Love, MD
> *Dr. Love's comprehensive and very helpful website includes a section on Internet myths about breast cancer.* www.susanlovemd.org

National Breast Cancer Coalition
> *Nation's largest breast cancer advocacy group dedicated to funding breast cancer research.* www.natlbcc.org

National Cancer Institute
> *The institute's Breast Cancer page, which includes information regarding clinical trials.* www.cancer.gov/cancertopics/types/breast

Think Before You Pink
> *A project of Breast Cancer Action, it's a resource for deciding how best to support nonprofit breastcancerrelated organizations.* www.thinkbeforeyoupink.org

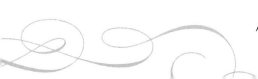

Women's Cancer Network
Information about breast cancer, therapies, and clinical trials.
www.wcn.org

Y-Me National Breast Cancer Organization
Dedicated to ensuring that no one goes through breast cancer alone, the organization offers a twenty-four-hour hotline for patients and their families at (800) 221-2141.
www.y-me.org

Young Survival Coalition
Resources for young women with breast cancer.
www.youngsurvival.org

DRESSING YOUR BREASTS

Books

Bra: A Thousand Years of Style, Support & Seduction, by Stephanie Pedersen (David & Charles, 2004). Fun and informative history of bras, including great movie star photos and how styles and shapes of brassieres evolved.

The Corset: A Cultural History, by Valerie Steele (Yale University Press, 2001). Gorgeous illustrated coffee-table book, with a complete history of the corset, confirming why this piece of boob dressing is still in fashion.

Dress Your Best: The Complete Guide to Finding the Style That's Right for Your Body, by Clinton Kelly and Stacy London (Three Rivers Press, 2005). Illustrations on how best to dress for your body type, be it for work, play, or evening.

The Lingerie Handbook, by Rebecca Apsan with Sarah Stark (Workman Publishing, 2006). Great resource for finding the right bra for your body type—together with many other intimate apparel suggestions.

Uplift: The Bra in America, by Jane Farrell-Beck and Colleen Gau (University of Pennsylvania Press, 2002). A complete and thorough history of bra manufacturing in America.

Sam Saboura's Real Style: Style Secrets for Real Women with Real Bodies, by Sam Saboura with L. G. Mansfield (Clarkson Potter, 2005). How to dress to enhance your shape and personal style.

What Not to Wear, by Trinny Woodall and Susannah Constantine
(Penguin Group, 2002). Specific style tips, with photos of authors—
one with bigger boobs and the other with smaller ones—providing
fashion advice for women with "big boobs" and "no boobs."

Websites
AA Lingerie
Online lingerie store dedicated to small-busted women.
www.aalingerie.com

Agent Provacateur
Hot lingerie, swimwear, and maternity bras.
www.agentprovocateur.com

Athleta
Good selection of sports bras and clothing for the active woman.
www.athleta.com

Bare Necessities
*Sexy lingerie and tips for men on how to buy women fabulous gifts. Bra sizes range
from 30A to 58C.*
www.barenecessities.com

Bella Materna Maternity Lingerie
*Luxurious nursing bras, maternity lingerie, and intimate apparel for pregnancy and
nursing.*
www.bellamaterna.com

The Big Bra Shop
From the UK, with sizes 28A–L to 56H.
www.thebigbrashop.com

Big Girls' Bras
In sizes 32AA to 50K.
www.biggerbras.com

Bra-Makers Supply
Everything you need to design your own bra, bustier, or swimsuit.
www.bramakers.com

Bra Smyth
Cups AA–H and everything in between, including swimwear.
www.brasmyth.com

Champion
Maker of the original jog bra.
www.championusa.com

Decent Exposures
Home of the "un-bra": all-cotton, made-to-order bras for everyone (girls, maternity, nursing) in sizes 30A to 54L.
www.decentexposures.com

Emily B. Maternity Wear
Beautiful bras and briefs for the expecting mum.
www.emily-b.co.uk

Enhancement Corporation of America
Breast forms and accessories for postmastectomy, lumpectomy, and enhancement needs.
www.enhancementcorp.com

Figleaves
Swimwear and bras from 28AA to 56FF.
www.figleaves.com

Frederick's of Hollywood
Bras, corsets, and very sexy lingerie.
www.fredericks.com/default.asp

Her Look Enterprises
Creators of nipple concealers (Low Beams), Take-Outs (for the better boob job), cleavage "Cupcakes," and "Matchsticks" to keep your clothes in place.
www.thebetterboobjob.com

House of Cadolle
Elegant bras and bustiers from the Parisian House of Cadolle.
www.cadolle.com/GB/accueil.shtml

Jodi Gallaer
Lingerie for full-busted women in sizes from 28C to 40H.
www.jodigallaer.com

Lands' End
Pick out custom swimsuits and shop for bras, including sizes up to 48DD.
www.landsend.com

La Petite Coquette
Exceptional lingerie from the author of The Lingerie Handbook, *Rebecca Apsan.*
www.thelittleflirt.com

L Straps
Bra straps you'll want to show off.
www.lstraps.com

Lula Lu
Website dedicated to smaller-size lingerie.
www.lulalu.com

Malia Mills Swimwear
Swimsuits in sizes 30A to 38DD and 2–16.
www.maliamills.com

Manhatten Wardrobe Supply
Home of Topstick Fashion-Fix double-sided tape and adhesive nonbra for plunging necklines.
www.wardrobesupplies.com/store/m2_clothestape.html#fashionfix

Nu Bra
The original no-straps, stick-on bra, including those that enhance the size of your breasts.
www.nubra.com

Title Nine
Sports bra choices for every breast type and activity.
www.titlenine.com

Twirlygirl.net
Extraordinary pasties for discriminating nipples.
www.twirlgirl.net

Victoria's Secret
Official website of Victoria's Secret, with bras, swimwear, and other sexy underthings.
www2.victoriassecret.com

Zovo Lingerie
The Boob Lady's hometown, favorite lingerie store.
www.zovolingerie.com

BREASTFEEDING

Books

The Breastfeeding Book: Everything You Need to Know About Nursing Your Child from Birth Through Weaning by Martha Sears, RN, and William Sears, MD (Little, Brown & Company, 2000). Comprehensive book on everything you need to know about breastfeeding.

The Nursing Mother's Companion by Kathleen Huggins, RM, MS (The Harvard Common Press, 2005). Helpful illustrated guidebook on the challenges and rewards of breastfeeding, with information on common problems and solutions.

The Womanly Art of Breastfeeding, 7th ed., La Leche League (Plume, 2004). One of the oldest and most comprehensive resources on breastfeeding.

Websites

Ameda
Information on breast pumps and accessories.
www.amedababy.com/?srcad=ameda-

Ask Dr. Sears
From the author of The Breastfeeding Book, *a great website where you can ask the doctor any questions you have about breastfeeding, nutrition, fussy babies, or childhood illnesses.*
www.askdrsears.com

Bosom Buddies
Nursing bras, clothes, and everything else for the nursing mom.
www.bosombuddies.com

The Breastchester
Stylish nursing clothes, nursing bras, breast pumps, et cetera.
www.breastchester.com

Breastfeeding.com
Maternity wear, resources, and humorous stories about beastfeeding.
www.breastfeeding.com

International Lactation Consultant Association
Worldwide organization with four thousand members in fifty countries.
www.ilca.org

The Lactivist
Supporting breastfeeding through humor with T-shirts and caps from the Reluctant Lactivist.
www.cafepress.com/thelactivist

La Leche League
The grandmother of all breastfeeding websites, includes lots of resources for new moms and a 24-hour nursing helpline.
www.lalecheleague.org

Maternity Mall
Includes many popular maternity and nursing clothing brands.
www.maternitymall.com/home.asp

Medela
Breastfeeding products and information from the breast pump manufacturer.
www.medela.com

National Alliance for Breastfeeding Advocacy
Dedicated to the protection and promotion of breastfeeding.
www.naba-breastfeeding.org

Nest Mom
Everything for the nursing mother, including bras and breastfeeding accessories.
www.nestmom.com

Promotion of Mother's Milk
List of breastfeeding links and information for employers on how to implement a supportive breastfeeding program.
www.promom.org

Unbuttoned Maternity
Stylish pregnancy and nursing clothes for the new mom.
www.unbuttonedmaternity.com

U.S. Breastfeeding Committee
Information and links to other breastfeeding resources.
www.usbreastfeeding.org

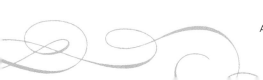

U.S. Department of Health and Human Services
Information on nursing, positions, and pumps and storage, and provides a helpful breastfeeding hotline at (800) 994-WOMAN, 9:00 AM–6:00 PM, Monday–Friday, EST.
www.4woman.gov/breastfeeding

Within Reach
Great breastfeeding pamphlet for mothers who wish to continue breastfeeding after they go back to work.
www.hmhbwa.org/forprof/materials/BCW_packet.htm

BREAST SURGERY

Books

The Breast Reconstruction Guidebook, by Kathy Steligo (Carlo Press, 2005). All about breast reconstruction after mastectomy.

Cosmetic Breast Surgery: A Complete Guide to Making the Right Decision from A to Double D, by Robert Freund with Alexander Van Dyne (Marlowe & Co., 2004). Comprehensive guide to numerous cosmetic breast surgery procedures, including discussion of patient expectations.

More Than Skin Deep: Exploring the Real Reasons Why Women Go Under the Knife, by Loren Eskenazi, MD, FACS, and Peg Streep (Harper Collins, 2007). Another perspective on why some women choose cosmetic surgery.

Reconstructing Aphrodite, by Terry Lorant and Dr. Loren Eskenazi (Verve Editions, 2001). A beautiful and inspiring nude photojournal of breast cancer survivors who have had reconstructive surgery.

The Smart Woman's Guide to Plastic Surgery: Essential Information from a Female Plastic Surgeon, by Jean M. Loftus, MD (McGraw-Hill, 2000). Handy checklists and personal stories about cosmetic breast augmentation and breast lift procedures.

Venus Envy: A History of Cosmetic Surgery, by Elizabeth Haiken (The John Hopkins University Press, 1997). Complete history of cosmetic surgery and the controversy about silicone breast implants.

*When Less Is More: The Complete Guide for Women Considering Breast Reduction
Surgery,* by Bethanne Snodgrass, MD, FACS (Harper Collins, 2005).
Everything you need to know about breast reduction surgery.

Your Complete Guide to Breast Reduction & Breast Lifts, by Alain Polynice, MD,
and Aloysius Smith, MD (Addicus Books, 2006). Illustrated guide
on choosing a surgeon and the risks and results of cosmetic breast
surgery (including use of implants).

Websites

American Society of Plastic Surgeons
*Official website of ASPS, including before and after photos, procedures, statistics, and
how to find a qualified plastic surgeon in your area.*
www.plasticsurgery.org

Breast Augmentation & Breast Implants Information
Website with personal stories about breast augmentation and implants.
www.implantinfo.com

Breast Implant Info
*Information on breast augmentation and reconstruction from the National Research
Center for Women & Families.*
www.breastimplantinfo.org

Myself Together Again
Breast reconstruction process and photos.
www.myselftogetheragain.org

Options for Women Seeking Breast Reconstruction
*Various reconstructive methods, what recovery is like, and what women can expect in
the way of results.*
www.mybreastreconstruction.com

RealSelf
*Information regarding cosmetic surgery procedures, with ratings and personal stories
from patients.*
www.realself.com

Talk Surgery, Inc.
Personal stories, before and after pictures, and forums on plastic surgery.
www.talksurgery.com

Publications

Harassment-Free Hallways, by the American Association of University Women. Guidebook on how to work toward stopping sexual harassment in schools.
www.aauw.org/ef/harass/pdf/completeguide.pdf.

Websites

The Bra Ball
> *What is made of 18,085 bras, stands five feet tall, and weighs 1,800 pounds?*
> www.braball.com

Burlesque Hall of Fame
> *A non-profit organization dedicated to promoting vintage burlesque. Sponsors the annual Ms. Exotic World event.*
> www.burlesquehall.com

Help My Flat Chest
> *Support and advice for the small breasted.*
> www.helpmyflatchest.com

Ms. Indigo Blue's Academy of Burlesque
> *Check out Ms. Indigo Blue's classes and learn how to take your own girls out for a spin!*
> www.academyofburlesque.com/

Skin Deep
> *The Environmental Working Group's website, where you can check out the safety of ingredients used in cosmetics and skin care products.*
> www.ewg.org/reports/skindeep

Notes

INTRODUCTION

1. PR Newswire. "Wacoal Study Reveals That 90 Million Women Are in the Wrong Size Bra, New York, May 20, 2005, found online at: www.prnewswire.com/cgi-bin/stories.

2. University of Michigan Comprehensive Cancer Center. "Women Overestimate Breast Cancer Risk, U-M Study Finds," June 7, 2005, found online at: www.cancer.med.umich.edu/news /breastcancerrisk05.shtml.

3. Kathryn M. Kah, Jimmie C. Holland, Marilyn S. Halper, and Daniel G. Miller, "Psychological Distress and Surveillance Behaviors of Women with a Family History of Breast Cancer," *JNCI Journal of the National Cancer Institute* 84, no. 1 (January 1992): 24-30; "Knowledge and Beliefs about Breast Cancer and Breast Self-Examination among Athletic and Nonathletic Women," *Nurs Res* 31, no. 6 (November–December 1981): 348-53; David J. Hil and Dace Shugg, "Breast Self-Examination Practices and Attitudes among Breast Cancer, Benign Breast Disease and General Practice Patients," *Health Education Research* 4, no. 2 (1989): 193-203; Strickland CJ, Feigl P, Upchurch C, et al. "Improving Breast Self-Examination Compliance: A Southwest Oncology Group Randomized Trial of Three Interventions." Preventative Medicine 26, no. 3 (May–June 1997): 320-32.

CHAPTER 1. BOSOM BUDDIES

1. Susan M. Love, *Dr. Susan Love's Breast Book,* 4th ed. revised (New York: De Capo Press, 2005), 3.

2. Elaine Morgan, *The Descent of Woman* (United Kingdom: Souvenir Press, 1985), 18.

3. Natalie Angier, *Woman: An Intimate Geography* (New York: Anchor Books, 2000), 151.

4. Ibid.

5. *The Descent of Woman,* 38.

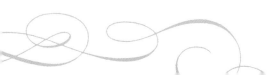

6. *Dr. Susan Love's Breast Book*, 4.

7. *Woman: An Intimate Geography*, 142.

8. Elissa Koff and Amy Benavage, "Breast Size Perception and Satisfaction, Body Image, and Psychological Functioning in Caucasian and Asian American College Women," *Sex Roles: A Journal of Research* 38, no. 7-8 (April 1998): 655-673.

9. Ibid.

10. Leora Pinhas, Breanda B. Toner, Alisha Ali, Paul Garfinkel, and Noreen Stuckless, "The Effects of the Ideal of Female Beauty on Mood and Body Satisfaction," *International Journal of Eating Disorders* 25, no. 2 (March 1999): 223-225.

11. Fiona Monro and Gail Huon, "Media-Portrayed Idealized Images, Body Shame, and Appearance Anxiety," *International Journal of Eating Disorders* 38, no. 1 (July 2005): 85-90.

12. Keira Knightley, "Shining Knightley," interview by Andrew Goldman, *Elle* (August 2006): 208.

13. Meema Spadola, *Breasts: Our Most Public Private Parts* (California: Wildcat Canyon Press, 1998), xv.

14. Desmond Morris, *The Naked Ape* (New York: Dell Publishing, 1957), 75.

15. Margo Maine, *Body Wars: Making Peace with Women's Bodies* (California: Gurze Books, 2000), 77.

16. James E. Maddux, ed., "Body Image, Mood, and Televised Images of Attractiveness: The Role of Social Comparison," by J. Cattarin, J. K. Thompson, T. Carmen, and W. Robyn, *Journal of Social and Clinical Psychology* 19, no. 2 (2000): 220-239.

17. Karyn Monget, "Booming with Boomers," *Women's Wear Daily* (February 26, 1996); Stephanie Thompson, "Bra Marketing Business Busts Out All Over," *Advertising Age* (April 20, 2006).

18. Fashion Industry Search Engine, "Dutch Women Buy Bigger Bras" (2006), found online at www.infomat.com/research/infreo000341 .html.

19. "Tempest in a D-Cup as Bust Sizes Grow," Tuesday, April 25, 2006, Reuters, Beijing.

20. Ibid.

21. Ibid.

22. Ibid.

23. *WordNet* 2.0, (c) 2003 Princeton University, found online at: http://wordnet.princeton.edu.

24. *Encyclopædia Britannica* (c) 2003.

25. Ibid.

26. www.urbandictionary.com.

27. Ibid.

28. Ibid.

29. Ibid.

30. www.georgecarlin.com/home/home.html.

31. www.urbandictionary.com.

32. Female Intelligence Agency, "Female Breasts: For Men or for Breastfeeding?" found online at www.007b.com.

CHAPTER 2. BRAS

1. Susan Nethero, "Oprah's Bra and Swimsuit Intervention," *The Oprah Winfrey Show,* May 20, 2005.

2. Victoria Roberts, proprietress of Zovo Lingerie, in a personal interview with the author June 27, 2005.

3. Karyn Monget, "Booming with Boomers," *Women's Wear Daily,* February 26, 1996.

4. Jane Farrell-Beck and Colleen Gau, *Uplift: The Bra in America* (Pennsylvania: University of Pennsylvania Press, 2002), 169.

5. Ibid., *xii.* Women held almost half of the more than 1,230 U.S. patents awarded for breast supporters between 1853 and 1969.

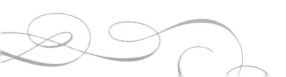

6. Valerie Steele, *The Corset: A Cultural History* (Connecticut: Yale University Press, 2001), 148.

7. Stephanie Pederson, *Bra: A Thousand Years of Style, Support & Seduction* (United Kingdom: David & Charles Publishing, 2004), 53.

8. Ibid., 103.

9. Bette Midler, *Mud Will Be Flung Tonight*, Atlantic Recording Corporation, 1985.

10. *Uplift: The Bra in America*, 18.

11. Ibid., 31-32.

12. *Bra: A Thousand Years of Style, Support & Seduction*, 32.

13. *Uplift: The Bra in America*, 24.

14. *Bra: A Thousand Years of Style, Support & Seduction*, 106.

15. Anne Casselman, "The Physics of . . . Bras," *Discover* magazine 26, no. 11 (November 2005): 19.

16. *Uplift: The Bra in America*, 164.

17. Ibid., 171.

18. Stephanie Thompson, "Bra Marketing Business Busts Out All Over," *Advertising Age,* April 20, 2006, found online at: http://adage.com/abstract.php?article_id=108633.

19. The NPD Group, "Market Insights on Women's Bras," http://retailindustry.about.com/b/a/113974.htm, September 9, 2004.

20. "Bra Marketing Business Busts Out All Over."

21. Jodi Gallaer, in a personal phone interview with the author, September 27, 2006.

22. Poupie Cadolle, in a personal email exchange with the author, April 3, 2007.

23. "The Physics of . . . Bras," page 18.

24. Rebecca Apsan, in a personal interview with the author, November 27, 2006.

25. Rebecca Apsan with Sarah Stark, *The Lingerie Handbook* (New York: Workman Publishing, 2006), 40.

26. Dr. Susan Love Research Foundation, "Common Breast Myths," found online at www.dslrf.org/rumors.html#3.

27. American Cancer Society, "Bras and Breast Cancer," found online at www.cancer.org/docroot/MED/content/MED_6_1x_Underwire_Bras.asp?sitearea=MED.

28. "Bra Masks Used to Ward off Sars," BBC News, May 9, 2003, found online at http://news.bbc.co.uk/1/hi/world/asia-pacific/3015219.stm.

CHAPTER 3. SPROUTING

1. Joan Jacobs Brumberg, *The Body Project: An Intimate History of American Girls* (New York: Vintage Books, 1997), 4.

2. Lynda Madaras with Area Madaras, *What's Happening to My Body? Book for Girls: A Growing Up Guide for Parents and Daughters* (New York: Newmarket Press, 2001), *xxxv*.

3. Dr. L. Kurt Midyett, Dr. Wayne V. Moore, and Dr. Jill D. Jacobson, "Are Pubertal Changes in Girls Before Age 8 Benign?" *Pediatrics* 111, no. 1 (January 2003): 47–51.

4. Dr. Paul B. Kaplowitz, Dr. Eric J. Slora, Dr. Richard C. Wasserman, Steven E. Pedlow, and Dr. Marcia E. Herman-Giddens, "Earlier Onset of Puberty in Girls: Relation to Increased Body Mass Index and Race," *Pediatrics* 108, no. 2 (August 2001): 347–353.

5. *The Body Project: An Intimate History of American Girls,* 4.

6. Marja Brandon, Seattle Girls' School, in a personal interview with the author, August 29, 2005.

7. *What's Happening to My Body? Book for Girls,* 204.

8. David Garner, "Survey Says: Body Image Poll Results," *Psychology Today,* February 1997.

9. Lisa M. Groesz, Michael P. Levine, and Sarah K. Murnen, "The Effect of Experimental Presentation of Thin Media Images on Body

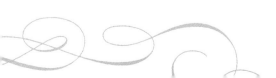

Satisfaction: A Meta-Analytic Review," *International Journal of Eating Disorders* 31, no.1 (January 2002).

10. *Dr. Susan Love's Breast Book,* 14.

11. *What's Happening to My Body? Book for Girls,* 32–35.

12. *Dr. Susan Love's Breast Book,* 14.

13. Softpedia, "Mark Wahlberg Not to Remove His Third Nipple," *Rolling Stone,* August 2005. Referenced online at: www.askmen.com /gossip/mark-wahlberg/wahlberg-keeps-third-nipple.html.

14. *Dr. Susan Love's Breast Book,* 59.

15. American Cancer Society, "Non-Cancerous Conditions," found online at www.cancer.org/docroot/CRI/content/CRI_2_6X_Non_ Cancerous_Breast_Conditions_59.asp?sitearea.

16. Ruth Bell, *Changing Bodies, Changing Lives* (New York: Three Rivers Press, 1998), 31.

17. *Dr. Susan Love's Breast Book,* 52.

18. Mattel press release, April 28, 2002, found online at www.shareholder.com/mattel/news/20020428-79086.cfm.

19. *Body Wars: Making Peace with Women's Bodies,* 210.

20. Helga Dittmar, Emma Halliwell, and Suzanne Ive, "Does Barbie Make Girls Want to Be Thin? The Effect of Experimental Exposure to Images of Dolls on the Body Image of 5- to 8-year-old Girls," *Developmental Psychology* 42, no. 2 (March 2006): 283–292.

21. *Body Wars: Making Peace with Women's Bodies,* 210.

22. Dr. David Radell and Dr. Zev Wanderer, *How Big Is Big? The Book of Sexual Measurements* (New York: Bell Publishing, 1982), 72–73.

23. *Body Wars: Making Peace with Women's Bodies,* 279.

24. Natalie Angier, "Drugs, Sports, Body Image and G.I. Joe," *The New York Times,* December 22, 1998.

25. *Uplift: The Bra in America,* 40, 71.

26. *The Body Project: An Intimate History of American Girls,* 112.

CHAPTER 4. TALKIN' TITS

1. Carolyn Latteier, *Breasts: The Women's Perspective on an American Obsession,* (New York: Haworth Press, 1998), 10.

2. "Breast Size Perception and Satisfaction, Body Image, and Psychological Functioning in Caucasian and Asian American College Women," 655-673.

3. Stacey Tantleff-Dunn, "Breast and Chest Size: Ideals and Stereotypes through the 1990s," *Sex Roles: A Journal of Research* 45, no. 3-4, (August 2001): 231-242.

4. *Breasts: The Women's Perspective on an American Obsession,* 10.

5. "Breast Size Perception and Satisfaction, Body Image, and Psychological Functioning in Caucasian and Asian American College Women," 655-673.

6. Ibid.

7. "Breast and Chest Size: Ideals and Stereotypes through the 1990s," 231-242.

8. Anthony H. Ahrens, James J. Gray, and Mia Foley Sypeck, "No Longer Just a Pretty Face: Fashion Magazines' Depictions of Ideal Female Beauty from 1959 to 1999," *International Journal of Eating Disorders* 36, no. 3 (November 2004): 342-347.

9. Dale L. Cusumano and J. Kevin Thompson, "Body Image and Body Shape Ideals in Magazines: Exposure, Awareness, and Internalization," *Sex Roles: A Journal of Research* 37 (November 1997): 701-721.

10. James J. Gray, Richard Leit, Harrison Pope Jr., "Cultural Expectations of Muscularity in Men: The Evolution of Playgirl Centerfolds," *International Journal of Eating Disorders* 29, no. 1 (January 2001): 90-93.

11. Stacey Tantleff-Dunn, "Biggest Isn't Always Best: The Effect of Breast Size on Perceptions of Women," *Journal of Applied Social Psychology* 32, no. 11 (November 2002): 2,253-2,265.

12. *Breasts: Our Most Public Private Parts*, 91.

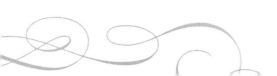

13. Sarah Katherine Lewis, in a personal interview with the author, January 1, 2007.

14. Elizabeth R. Didie and David B. Sarwer, "Factors that Influence the Decision to Undergo Cosmetic Breast Augmentation Surgery," *Journal of Women's Health* 12, no. 3 (April 2003): 241–253.

15. Elizabeth R. Didie and David B. Sarwer, "Factors that Influence the Decision to Undergo Cosmetic Breast Augmentation Surgery," *Journal of Women's Health* 12, no. 3 (April 2003): 241–253.

16. www.plasticsurgery.com.

17. "A Retrospective Study of Changes in Physical Symptoms and Body Image after Reduction Mammaplasty", Glatt, Brian S. MD; Sarwer, David B. PhD; O'Hara, Daniel E. MD; Hamori, Christine MD; Bucky, Louis PMD; LaRossa, Don MD, *Plastic & Reconstructive Surgery,* 103(1):76:82, January 1999.

18. Title VII of the 1964 Civil Rights Act. 42 U.S.C. 2000e-2, found online at: http://www.law.cornell.edu/uscode /html/uscode42/usc_sec_42_00002000---e000-.html.

19. U.S. Equal Employment Opportunity Commission, "Sexual Harassment," February 2007, found at www.eeoc.gov/types/sexual _harassment.html.

20. "Hostile Hallways: Bullying, Teasing, and Sexual Harassment in School," American Association of University Women, 2001, found online at www.aauw.org/research/girls_education/hostile.cfm.

21. "Children Online: Statistics," CyberAngels, 2005, www.cyberangels .org/statistics.html.

22. Marcella Fleming-Reed, in a personal phone interview with the author, March 20, 2007.

23. "About Hooters," found online at www.hooters .com/company/about_hooters.

24. "Hooters Girl Legal Acknowledgment," found online at www.thesmokinggun.com/archive/091505-1hooters8.html.

25. *HI Ltd. Partnership vs. Winghouse* or Florida, No. 6;a03-cv-116-Orl-22JGG (M.D. Fla. 2004).

26. *Breasts: Our Most Public Private Parts*, 101.

CHAPTER 5. UNFETTERED BREASTS

1. Marilyn Yalom, *A History of the Breast* (New York: Ballentine Books, 1997), 3.

2. *A History of the Breast*, 122.

3. "Curtains for Semi-Nude Justice Statue," January 2002, *BBC News Online,* http://news.bbc.co.uk/2/hi/americas/1788845.stm.

4. *Breasts: The Women's Perspective on an American Obsession*, 158.

5. La Leche League International, *La Leche League International 2004-2005 Annual Report,* www.lalecheleague.org/docs/05_LLLI_AR.pdf.

6. Ruowei Li, Jason Hsia, Fred Fridinger, Abeda Hussain, Sandra Benton-Davis, and Laurence Grummer-Strawn, "Public Beliefs about Breastfeeding Policies in Various Settings," *Journal of The American Dietetic Association* 104, no. 7 (July 2004): 1,162-1,168.

7. Ruowei Li, Valerie J. Rock, and Laurence Grummer-Strawn, "Changes in Public Attitudes toward Breastfeeding in the United States, 1999-2003," *Journal of the American Dietetic Association* 107, no. 1 (January 2007): 122-127.

8. Melissa R. Vance, "Breastfeeding Legislation in the United States: A General Overview and Implications for Helping Mothers," found online at www.lalecheleague.org/llleaderweb/LV/LVJunJul05p51.html.

9. "The Bikini Passes the Half-Century Mark," CNN, July 5, 1996, found online at www.cnn.com/STYLE/9607/06/bikini.aniversary.

10. *Uplift: The Bra in America*, 147-148.

11. Sophia Banay, "Top Topless Beaches 2006," *Forbes,* January 13, 2006, found online at: www.forbes.com/2006/01/12/topless-beaches-resorts-cx_sb_0113feat_ls.html.

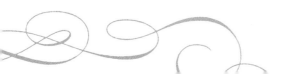

12. Federation of Canadian Naturists, "Women's Top-Free Rights Entrenched in Ontario," December 1996, found online at www.fcn.ca/Gwen.html.

13. Court of Appeal for Ontario, "Her Majesty the Queen vs. Gwen Jacob," found online at www.canlii.org/on/cas/onca/1996/1996onca10568.html.

14. Dr. Paul Rapoport, coordinator of TERA, in a personal phone interview with the author, December 13, 2006.

15. A History of the Breast, 244.

16. Jessica Werner, "God's Better Half Just Woke Up, and Boy Is She Mad," San Francisco Chronicle, June 22, 2006; author blog at www.breastsnotbombs.blogspot.com.

17. Robyn Read, "Play Launches Calendar for Breast of Canada," found online at www.breastofcanada.com/media/031004-merc.html.

18. Trade Association for Nude Recreation, "Your Clothing Optional Getaway Awaits You," found online at www.tanr.com/main.php.

19. Bernard Sobel, A Pictorial History of Burlesque (New York: Crown Publishers, 1956).

20. Ms. Indigo Blue, in personal interview with the author, November 26, 2006.

21. www.exoticworldusa.org.

22. www.teaseorama.com.

23. Claire Hoffman, "Baby, Give Me a Kiss," The Los Angeles Times, August 8, 2006; Vanessa Grigoriadis, "Wild Thing," Rolling Stone, May 22, 2002.

CHAPTER 6. MAMMARIES IN MOTION

1. www.shockabsorber.co.uk/uk/index.asp?page+13.

2. Bruce R. Maron, Kelly-Ann Page, and Keiron Fallon, "An Analysis of Movement and Discomfort of the Female Breast During Exercise and the Effects of Breast Support," Journal of Science and Medicine in Sports 2, no. 2 (June 1999): 134-144.

3. K. A. Bowles, J. R. Steele, and R. Chaunchaiyakul, "Do Current Sports Brassiere Designs Impede Respiratory Function?" *Medicine & Science in Sports & Exercise* 37, no. 9 (September 2005): 1,633–1,640.

4. S. A. Maha Abdel Hadi, "Sports Brassiere: Is It a Solution for Mastalgia?" *The Breast Journal* 6, no. 6 (November/December 2000): 407.

5. Malia Mills Swimwear: www.maliamills.com.

6. Bruce Horovitz, "Swimsuit Buyers Leap for High-Tech, Versatile Styles," *USA Today,* May 27, 2004.

7. Barbara L. Frederickson, Tomi-Ann Roberts, Stephanie M. Noll, Diane M. Quinn, and Jean M. Twenge, "That Swimsuit Becomes You: Sex Differences in Self-Objectification, Restrained Eating, and Math Performance," *Journal of Personality and Social Psychology* 75, no. 1 (July 1998): 269–284.

8. Fiona Monro and Gail Huon, "Media-Portrayed Idealized Images, Body Shame, and Appearance Anxiety," *The International Journal of Eating Disorders* 38, no. 1 (July 2005): 85–90.

9. Leora Pinhas, Brenda B. Toner, Alisha Ali, Paul E. Garfinkel, and Noreen Stuckless, "The Effects of the Ideal of Female Beauty on Mood and Body Satisfaction," *The International Journal of Eating Disorders* 25, no. 2 (March 1999): 223–226.

10. NPDFashionworld Survey, January 23, 2002, found online at: www.npd.com/press/releases/press_020123.htm.

11. www.landsend.com.

12. Kate Starbird, in a personal interview with the author, November 7, 2006.

13. "The Physics of . . . Bras," page 18.

14. "An Analysis of Movement and Discomfort of the Female Breast During Exercise and the Effects of Breast Support," 134–144.

15. *Uplift: The Bra in America,* 31.

16. K. A. Page and J. R. Steele, "Breast Motion and Sports Brassiere Design: Implications for Future Research," *Sports Medicine* 27, no. 44 (April 1999): 205–211.

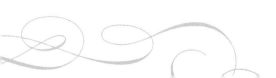

17. Michael F. Roizen, MD, and Mehmet C. Oz, MD, *You: The Owner's Manual,* (New York: Harper Collins, 2005), 50.

18. Joan Pagano, *Strength Training for Women* (New York: Dorling Kindersley Publishing, 2002), 15.

19. Shirley Archer, *Busting Out: Putting Your Best Breasts Forward,* (New York: Chronicle Books, 2007), 42.

CHAPTER 7. FULLY EMPLOYED BOOBS

1. Martha Sears, RM, and William Sears, MD, *The Breastfeeding Book* (New York: Little, Brown & Company, 2000), 10.

2. American Academy of Pediatrics Policy Statement, "Breastfeeding and the Use of Human Milk," *Pediatrics* 115, no. 2 (February 2005): 497.

3. *The Breastfeeding Book,* 24.

4. "Breastfeeding and the Use of Human Milk," 499.

5. "Position of the American Dietetic Association: Promoting and Supporting Breastfeeding," *Journal of the American Dietetic Association* 105, no. 5 (May 2005): 716-717; found online at www.adajournal .org/article/PIIS0002822305003299/abstract.

6. Ibid.

7. *The Breastfeeding Book,* 238.

8. www.kathydettwyler.org.

9. www.unicef.org/programme/brastfeeding/baby.htm.

10. www.babyfriendlyusa.org.

11. *The Breastfeeding Book,* 36.

12. Judy Harrigel, ILCA, during a phone interview with the author, February 27, 2007.

13. Paula Meier, Linda Brown, Nancy Hurst, Diane Spatz, Janet Engstrom, Lynn Borucki, and Ann Krouse, "Nipple Shields for Preterm Infants: Effect on Milk Transfer and Duration of Breastfeeding," *Journal of Human Lactation* 16, no. 2 (2000): 105-114.

14. Kathleen Huggins, RM, MS, *Nursing Mother's Companion* (Boston: The Harvard Common Press, 2005), 141.

15. A. Pisacane and P. Continisio, "Breastfeeding and Perceived Changes in the Appearance of the Breasts: A Retrospective Study," *Acta Paediatrica* 93, no. 10 (October 2004): 1,346–1,348.

16. *Dr. Susan Love's Breast Book,* 20.

17. *The Breastfeeding Book,* 63.

18. Geoff Der, G. David Batty, and Ian Deary, "Effect of Breast Feeding on Intelligence in Children: Prospective Study, Sibling Pairs Analysis, and Meta-Analysis," *British Medical Journal* 333, no. 7575 (November 2006): 945.

19. *Dr. Susan Love's Breast Book,* 16.

20. Anne Diamond, cofounder Bella Materna, in a personal interview with the author, October 2, 2006.

CHAPTER 8. LOVERS LOVE 'EM

1. *Breasts: The Women's Perspective on an American Obsession,* 158.

2. *How Big Is Big? The Book of Sexual Measurements,* 160; found online at: www.kinseyinstitute.org/research/ak-data.html.

3. Alfred Kinsey, The Kinsey Institute, data from Alfred Kinsey's studies, found online at www.kinseyinstitute.org/research/ak-data .html.

4. *How Big Is Big? The Book of Sexual Measurements,* 162.

5. Cindy Meston and Roy Levin, "Nipple/Breast Stimulation and Sexual Arousal in Young Men and Women," *The Journal of Sexual Medicine* 3, no. 3 (May 2006): 450–454.

6. Conservative talkshow radio host Rush Limbaugh admitted his addiction to prescription drugs on a nationally syndicated show, October 10, 2003. See: "Limbaugh Admits Addiction to Pain Medication," October 10, 2003, CNN.com.

7. "Hormone Involved in Reproduction May Have Role in the Maintenance of Relationships," UCSF, July 14, 1999, found online at www.oxytocin.org/oxytoc/index.html.

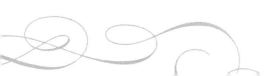

8. J. A. Amico and B. E. Finley, "Breast Stimulation in Cycling Women, Pregnant Women and a Woman with Induced Lactation: Pattern of Release of Oxytocin, Prolactin and Luteinizing Hormone," *Clinical Endocrinol* 25, no. 2 (August 1986): 97-106.

9. K. Christensson, B. A. Nilsson, S. Stock, A. S. Matthiesen, and K. Uvnas-Moberg, "Effect of Nipple Stimulation on Uterine Activity and on Plasma Levels of Oxytocin in Full Term, Healthy, Pregnant Women," *Acta obstetricia et gynecologica Scandinavica* 68, no. 3 (1989): 206-209.

10. www.kinseyinstitute.org/research/ak-data.html.

11. Dr. Miriam Stoppard, *101 Essential Tips: Breast Care* (New York: Dorling Kindersley Publishing, 1997), 26.

12. *How Big Is Big? The Book of Sexual Measurements*, 150.

13. *101 Essential Tips: Breast Care*, 26-27.

14. Stefan Bechtel, Laurence R. Stains, and the editors of *Men's Health, Sex: A Man's Guide* (New York: Berkley Press, 1998), 109.

15. Terry Lorant, photographer, *Reconstructing Aphrodite,* (New York: Syracuse University Press, 2001).

16. Ibid., 58.

17. Dolf Zillmann, Jennigs Bryant (1988) "Pornography's Impact on Sexual Satisfaction," Journal of Applied Social Psychology 18(5): 438-453.

18. Rachel Kramer Bussel, "Meet the Boobiesexuals," *The Village Voice,* March 24, 2006.

19. *The Lingerie Handbook,* 144.

20. *How Big Is Big? The Book of Sexual Measurements,* 223.

21. UPI, April 20, 2004: www.accessmylibrary.com/coms2/summary_0286-7049184_ITM.

CHAPTER 9. YOUR BREAST POTENTIAL

1. American Cancer Society, "Sunlight and Ultraviolet Exposure," found online at www.cancer.org/docroot/PED/content/ped_7_1_ What_You_Should_Know_About_Ultraviolet_Exposure .asp?sitearea=&level=.

2. Dr. Miriam Stoppard, *Breast Health* (New York: DK Publishing, Inc., 1998), 38.

3. Robert M. Freund, MD, *Cosmetic Breast Surgery: A Complete Guide to Making the Right Decision—from A to Double D* (New York: Marlowe & Co., 2004), 21-23; FDA Consumer, "Quackery Targets Teens," April 1990 update, found at www.cfsan.fda.gov/~dms/qa-qak2.html.

4. www.mybrava.com/breast-health-and-options.asp.

5. http://home.comcast.net/~drmomentum/bravargh/Forum /Forum.html.

6. Robert M. Freund, MD, FACS, with Alexander Van Dyne, *Cosmetic Breast Surgery: A Complete Guide to Making the Right Decision—from A to Double D* (New York: Marlowe & Company, 2004), 25.

7. *Busting Out: Putting Your Best Breasts Forward,* 43.

8. http://lalecheleague.org/lllleaderweb/Lv/LVJunJul99p64html.

9. Anne McTiernan, Julie Gralow, and Lisa Talbott, *Breast Fitness: An Optimal Exercise and Health Plan for Reducing Your Risk of Breast Cancer* (New York: St. Martin's, 2000), 7.

10. American Cancer Society, *Surveillance Research: Breast Cancer Facts & Figures 2005-2006* (Atlanta: American Cancer Society, Inc., 2005).

11. Centers for Disease Control, "Leading Causes of Death, Females—United States, 2003," found online at www.cdc.gov/cancer/breast/statistics.

12. Michelle Althuis, Jaclyn Dozier, William Anderson, Susan Devesa, and Louise Brinton, "Global Trends in Breast Cancer Incidence and Mortality 1973-1997," *International Journal of Epidemiology* 34, no. 2 (2005): 405-412.

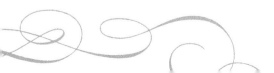

13. http://seer.cancer.gov/statfacts/html/breast.html.

14. American Cancer Society, "What Are the Risk Factors for Breast Cancer?" found online at www.cancer.org/docroot/CRI/content /CRI_2_4_2X_What_are_the_risk_factors_for_breast_cancer _5.asp?sitearea=.

15. http://seer.cancer.gov/statfacts/html/breast.html.

16. *Dr. Susan Love's Breast Book,* 326-327.

17. "What Are the Risk Factors for Breast Cancer?" www.cancer.org /docroot/CRI/content/CRI_2_4_2X_What_are_the_risk_ factors_for_breast_cancer_5.asp?sitearea=.

18. Norman F. Boyd, Helen Guo, Lisa J. Martin, Limei Sun, Jennifer Stone, Eve Fishell, Roberta A. Jong, Greg Hislop, Anna Chiarelli, Salomon Minkin, and Martin J. Yaffe, "Mammographic Density and the Risk and Detection of Breast Cancer," *The New England Journal of Medicine* 356, no. 3 (January 2007): 227-236.

19. Ibid.

20. Mark Clemons and Paul Goss, "Estrogen and the Risk of Breast Cancer," *The New England Journal of Medicine* 344, no. 4 (January 2001): 276-285.

21. Zora Brown, LaSalle D. Lefall, Jr, with Elizabeth Platt, *100 Questions & Answers about Breast Cancer* (Sudbury, MA: Jones & Bartlett, 2003), 25.

22. Dr. Constance Lehman, in a personal interview with the author, September 27, 2006.

23. "What Are the Risk Factors for Breast Cancer?" www.cancer.org /docroot/CRI/content/CRI_2_4_2X_What_are_the_risk_factors _for_breast_cancer_5.asp?sitearea=.

24. Ibid.

25. Jennifer Wilder, MD, "Women Most Fear Breast Cancer, but Heart Disease Is the Top Killer," Society for Women's Health Research, July 14, 2005, found online at www.womenshealthresearch.org/site /News2?page=NewsArticle&id=5361&news_iv_ctrl=0&abbr=press.

26. "New Survey Shows Nearly 50 Percent of Women Over 40 Do Not Receive Recommended Annual Mammogram," February 15, 2007. Press Release from Eastman Kodak Company, found online at: http://press-releases.techwhack.com/7547/new-survey-shows-nearlt-50-percent.

27. "For Women Facing a Breast Biopsy," www.cancer.org/docroot/CRI/content/CRI_2_4_6x_For_Women_Facing_a_Breast_Biopsy.asp.

28. "Benefits and Risks of Mammography," found online at www.imaginis.com/breasthealth/mammo_benefit-risk.asp.

29. Indraneel Mittra, Michael Baum, Hazel Thornton, and Joan Houghton, "Is Clinical Breast Examination an Acceptable Alternative to Mammographic Screening?" *BMJ* 321, no. 7,268 (200): 1,071–1,073, found online at www.bmj.com/cgi/content/full/bmj;321/7268/1071.

30. *Dr. Susan Love's Breast Book,* 235.

31. *Breast Fitness: An Optimal Exercise and Health Plan for Reducing Your Risk of Breast Cancer,* 40.

32. www.imaginis.com/breasthealth/bcmyths.asp.

33. National Cancer Institute website: www.cancer.gov/cancertopics/wyntk/breast/page6.

34. www.cancer.gov/newscenter/pressreleases/DMISTrelease.

35. National Cancer Institute: www.cancer.gov/cancertopics/factsheet/detection/screening-mammograms.

36. www.medicare.gov/health/mammography.asp.

37. www.cancer.gov/newscenter/pressreleases/DMISTFastFacts.

38. American Cancer Society: www.cancer.org/docroot/PED/content/PED_2_3X_Mammography_and_Other_Breast_Imaging_Procedures.asp?sitearea=PED.

39. American Cancer Society, "Mammograms and Other Breast Imaging Procedures," found online at www.cancer.org/docroot/PED/content/PED_2_3X_Mammography_and_Other_Breast_Imaging_Procedures.asp?sitearea=PED.

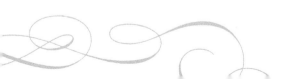

40. Ibid.

41. Samantha King, *Pink Ribbons, Inc.: Breast Cancer and the Politics of Philanthropy* (Minneapolis: University of Minnesota Press, 2006).

CHAPTER 10. IN SICKNESS AND IN HEALTH

1. American Cancer Society, *Breast Cancer Facts & Figures 2006-2006* (Atlanta: American Cancer Society), 10-11.

2. "For Women Facing a Breast Biopsy," www.cancer.org/docroot/CRI /content/CRI_2_4_6x_For_Women_Facing_a_Breast_Biopsy.asp.

3. C. A. Gateley and R. E. Mansel, "Management of Cyclical Breast Pain," *British Journal of Hospital Medicine* 43, no. 5 (May 1990): 330-332.

4. *Dr. Susan Love's Breast Book*, 61.

5. *Breast Health*, 27.

6. Antonino Millet and Frederick Dirbas, "Clinical Management of Breast Pain: A Review," *Obstetrical & Gynecological Survey* 57, no. 7 (July 2002): 451-461.

7. "Sports Brassiere: Is It a Solution for Mastalgia?": 407-409.

8. American Cancer Society, Cancer Reference Information, "Benign Breast Conditions," found online at www.cancer.org/docroot/CRI /content/CRI_2_6X_Benign_Breast_Conditions_59.asp.

9. *Dr. Susan Love's Breast Book*, 87-90.

10. "Benign Breast Conditions," www.cancer.org/docroot/CRI/content /CRI_2_6X_Benign_Breast_Conditions_59.asp.

11. Ibid.

12. American Medical Association, *Complete Medical Encyclopedia* (New York: Random House, 2003), 828.

13. *Breast Fitness: An Optimal Exercise and Health Plan for Reducing Your Risk of Breast Cancer*, 3-4.

14. American Cancer Society, *Cancer Facts & Figures 2007* (Atlanta: American Cancer Society), 4.

15. "For Women Facing a Breast Biopsy," www.cancer.org/docroot /CRI/content/CRI_2_4_6x_For_Women_Facing_a_Breast _Biopsy.asp.

16. Virgnia L. Ernster, John Barclay, Karla Kerlikowske, Heather Wilkie, and Rachel Ballard-Barbash, "Mortality Among Women with Ductal Carcinoma In Situ," *Archives of Internal Medicine* 160, no. 7 (April 2000): 953-958.

17. *Breast Fitness,* 25-26; *Dr. Susan Love's Breast Book,* 264.

18. James S. Olson, *Bathsheba's Breast: Women, Cancer and History* (Baltimore, The John Hopkins University Press, 2002), 10.

19. Barron H. Lerner, MD, *The Breast Cancer Wars: Fear, Hope, and the Pursuit of a Cure in Twentieth-Century America* (New York: Oxford University Press, 2001).

20. Ibid.

21. Ibid.

22. The Women's Health and Cancer Rights Act of 1998 (WHCRA), www.dol.gov/ebsa/Publications/whcra.html.

23. American Cancer Society. *Cancer Facts & Figures 2007.* Atlanta: American Cancer Society; 20071, 1124. American Cancer Society, "Living with Lymphedema," May 12, 1998.

24. Ronit Elk, PhD, and Monica Morrow, MD, *Breast Cancer for Dummies* (Wiley Publishing, 2003), 163.

25. Ronit Elk, PhD, and Monica Morrow, MD, *Breast Cancer for Dummies* (Wiley Publishing, 2003), 163.

26. American Cancer Society. *Breast Cancer Facts & Figures 2005-2006.* Atlanta: American Cancer Society, Inc., 8.

27. *Breast Cancer Facts & Figures 2005-2006* (Atlanta: American Cancer Society), 8.

28. Ibid.

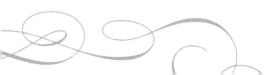

29. Yvonne Lee, "Breast Reconstruction Rates Remain Low Despite Law Mandating Coverage of Surgery," *All Headline News,* January 25, 2006.

30. Caprice K. Christian, MD, et al., "A Multi-Institutional Analysis of the Socioeconomic Determinants of Breast Reconstruction," *Annals of Surgery* 243, no. 2 (2006): 241-249.

CHAPTER 11. CUT AND PASTE

1. *Dr. Susan Love's Breast Book,* 40.

2. Michael Ciaschini, MD, "History of Plastic Surgery," found online at www.emedicine.com/plastic/topic433.htm.

3. Elizabeth Haiken, *Venus Envy: The History of Cosmetic Surgery* (Maryland: The John Hopkins University Press, 1997), 4.

4. The American Society for Aesthetic Plastic Surgery, February 2006 Consumer Survey.

5. American Academy of Cosmetic Surgery, 2006 Consumer Perception Survey, September 13, 2006, press release.

6. American Society of Plastic Surgeons, www.plasticsurgery.org.

7. Ibid.

8. Gynecomastia is a condition in which a man grows femalelike breasts, most commonly due to a hormonal imbalance.

9. American Society of Plastic Surgeons, www.plasticsurgery.org.

10. Valerie J. Ablaza, MD, and Allen D. Rosen, MD, *Beauty in Balance: A Common Sense Approach to Cosmetic Surgery and Treatments* (New York: MD Publish 2006), 22.

11. Canice E. Crerand, Martin E. Franklin, and David B. Sarwer, "Body Dysmorphic Disorder and Cosmetic Surgery," *Plastic and Reconstructive Surgery* 118, no. 7 (December 2006): 167e-180e.

12. *Beauty in Balance: A Common Sense Approach to Cosmetic Surgery and Treatments,* 17.

13. www.tit4tat.net.

14. Associated Press, "Tyra Banks Proves Her Breasts Are Real," September 21, 2005, found online at www.msnbc.msn.com/id/9427670.

15. Paul Joannides, *Guide to Getting It On* (Oregon: Goofy Foot Press, 2006), 441.

16. Anne Slowey, "Elle Fashion Know-It-All: Size Matters," *Elle Magazine,* February 2007, 80.

17. The Boston Women's Health Book Collective, *Our Bodies, Ourselves* (New York: Touchstone, 2005), 5.

18. Daniel J. DeNoon, "Breast Implants Lift Sex, Self-Esteem," Web MD Medical News, March 23, 2007, found online at www.webmd.com/skin-beauty/news/20070323/breast-implants-lift-sex-self-esteem.

19. Alex Kuczyncki, *Beauty Junkies: Inside Our $15 Billion Obsession with Cosmetic Surgery* (New York: Doubleday, 2006), 246.

20. Nancy Etcoff, *Survival of the Prettiest: The Science of Beauty* (New York: Anchor Books, 2000), 242.

21. American Academy of Cosmetic Surgery, 2006 Consumer Perception Survey Results, September 13, 2006.

22. David B. Sarwer, Leanne Magee, and Vicki Clark, "Physical Appearance and Cosmetic Medical Treatments: Physiological and Socio-Cultural Influences," *Journal of Cosmetic Dermatology* 2, no. 1 (January 2003): 29.

23. Jonathan Heidt, *The Happiness Hypothesis: Finding Modern Truth in Ancient Wisdom* (New York: Basic Books, 2006), 93.

24. Cynthia Figueroa-Haas, PhD, "Effect of Breast Augmentation Mammoplasty on Self-Esteem and Sexuality: A Quantitative Analysis," *Plastic Surgical Nursing* 27 (January/March 2007): 16–36.

25. *Venus Envy: The History of Cosmetic Surgery,* 232–233.

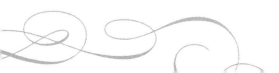

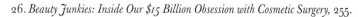

26. *Beauty Junkies: Inside Our $15 Billion Obsession with Cosmetic Surgery,* 255.

27. *Venus Envy: The History of Cosmetic Surgery,* 236.

28. Dr. Judith Reichman, "Woman with Fake Boobs Has Real Health Worries," MSNBC, May 26, 2006, found online at: www.msnbc.msn.com/id/12991972.

29. *Beauty Junkies: Inside Our $15 Billion Obsession with Cosmetic Surgery,* 255.

30. Nicole Cummings, ImplantInfo.com, www.implantinfo.com /media.htm.

31. Reuters Health, "Breast Implants Linked to Suicide, but Not Cancer," August 18, 2005, found online at: www. upmccancercenters.com/news/reuters/reuters.cfm?article=7970.

32. Reuters Health, "Breast Implants Linked Again with Suicide Risk," April 13, 2006, found online at www.upmccancercenters .com/news/reuters/reuters.cfm?article=7970.

33. Dr. Drew Welk, in a personal interview with the author, October 4, 2005.

34. Nicole Cummings, ImplantInfo.com, www.implantinfo.com/ media.htm.

35. Susan Seligson, *Stacked: A 32DDD Reports from the Front* (New York: Bloomsbury, 2007), 111.

36. American Society of Plastic Surgeons, "Cosmetic Plastic Surgery 'Mommy Makeovers' on the Rise," March 22, 2007, found online at www.plasticsurgery.org/media/press_releases/2006 -Stats-Mommy-Makeover.cfm.

37. www.myfreeimplants.com/about_us.asp.

38. *Beauty Junkies: Inside Our $15 Billion Obsession with Cosmetic Surgery,* 264.

39. "Fake Boobs Are a 'Turn-Off' for Men," found online at http://news.sawf.org/lifestyle/23840.aspx; www.ananova.com /news/story/sm_2031005.html.

40. Mister Poll: Breasts Real or Fake? Guys: Breast Size Poll, found online at: www.misterpoll.com/results.mpl?id=1903416511; www.misterpoll.com/results.mpl?id=275696572.

41. "What Men Think about Breast Implants," found online at www.implantforum.com/men.html.

42. Jim Bauer, "How to: Differentiate Real from Fake Breasts," found online at www.askmen.com/fashion /how_to_200/246_how_to.html.

43. Tom Chiarella, "How Men Really Feel about Breast Implants," *O, The Oprah Magazine* (July 2006): 122.

44. Ibid.

45. *Cosmetic Breast Surgery: A Complete Guide to Making the Right Decision,* 74.

46. Ibid., 29.

47. Jean M. Loftus, MD, *The Smart Woman's Guide to Plastic Surgery: Essential Information from a Female Plastic Surgeon* (New York: McGraw Hill, 2000), 122.

48. *Dr. Susan Love's Breast Book,* 42.

49. Salynn Boyles, "Most Don't Rebuild Breast After Cancer," WebMDHealth, January 27, 2006.

50. Dr. Drew Welk, in a personal interview with the author, October 4, 2005.

51. Kathy Steligo, *Breast Reconstruction Guidebook: Issues and Answers from Research to Recovery* (California: Carlo Press, 2005), 18-19.

52. Albert Losken, Inessa Fishman, Donald Denson, Hunter Moyer, and Grant Carlson, "An Objective Evaluation of Breast Symmetry and Shape Differences Using 3-Dimensional Images," *Annals of Plastic Surgery* 55 (December 2005): 571-575.

53. John Stossel, ABC News Commentary, June 24, 2005, found online at http://abcnews.go.com /2020/Health/ story?id=875821&page=1.

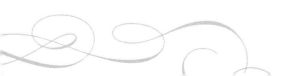

54. www.hilary.com/features/teen-breast-implants.html.

55. "Cosmetic Surgery Age Distribution," American Society of Plastic Surgeons, 2006.

56. Policy Statement, "Breast Augmentation in Teenagers," American Society of Plastic Surgeons, December 2004.

57. *Venus Envy: The History of Cosmetic Surgery,* 35.

58. Ibid., 249.

59. Ibid., 278.

60. Ibid., 232.

61. *Dr. Susan Love's Breast Book,* 44.

62. NBC, MSNBC, "Ban on Silicone Breast Implants Lifted," November 17, 2006, found online at www.msnbc.msn.com/id/15770935.

63. Eric Wilson, "Fashion Refigured," *The New York Times,* May 12, 2005.

64. American Society of Plastic Surgeons, "Regional Distribution, Cosmetic Procedures," 2006.

CHAPTER 12. THE MORE MATURE BREAST

1. Centers for Disease Control, "Trends in Aging—United States and Worldwide, 2003," found online at www.cdc.gov/mmwr/preview/mmwrhtml/mm5206a2.htm.

2. AARP Foundation Women's Leadership Circle Study, "Looking at Act II of Women's Lives: Thriving & Striving from 45 On," found online at www.aarp.org/research/housing-mobility/indliving/wlcresearch.html.

3. National Alliance on Mental Illness, Women and Depression, November 2003, www.nami.org.

4. Susan A. Sabatino, MD, "Breast Cancer Risk and Provider Recommendation for Mammography among Recently Unscreened Women in the United States," *Journal of General Internal Medicine* 21, no. 4 (April 2006): 285.

5. Christiane Northrup, MD, *The Wisdom of Menopause: Creating Physical and Emotional Health During the Change,* revised ed. (New York: Bantam Books, 2006), 437-438.

6. *Breast Health,* 11.

7. Marilynn Marchione, "Breast Cancer Rate Plunged 7 Percent in '03," December 14, 2006, found online at http://www.foxnews.com/wires/2006Dec14/0,4670,BreastCancer,00.html.

8. M. M. McNicholas, J. P. Heneghan, M. H. Milner, T. Tunney, J. B. Hourihane, and D. P. MacErlaine, "Pain and Increased Mammographic Density in Women Receiving Hormone Replacement Therapy: A Prospective Study," *American Journal of Roentgenology* 163, no. 2 (August 1994): 311-316; P. A. Carney, D. L. Miglioretti, B. C. Yankaskas, K. Kerlikowske, R. Rosenberg, C. M. Rutter, B. M. Geller, L. A. Abraham, S. H. Taplin, M. Dignan, G. Cutter, and R. Ballard-Barbash, "The Effects of Age, Breast Density, and Hormone Therapy on the Accuracy of Screening Mammograms," *Annals of Internal Medicine* 138, no. 3 (February 2003): 1-28.

9. *The Wisdom of Menopause,* 141.

10. Yale–New Haven Hospital, "Strength Training Boon for Aging Women," July 30, 2002, found online at www.ynhh.org/healthlink/womens/womens_7_02.html.

11. M. E. Nelson, M. A. Fiatarone, C. M. Morganti, I. Trice, R. A. Greenberg, and W. J. Evans, "Effects of High-Intensity Strength Training on Multiple Risk Factors of Osteoporotic Fractures," *JAMA* 272, no. 24 (December 1994): 1909-14.

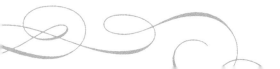

Index

A

action figures, 54
anatomical characteristics, 7-9
Anderson, Pamela, 65
Apsan, Rebecca, 30, 32, 148
Archer, Shirley, 114, 158
areola, 8, 89, 117, 214
artistic works, 90
Ashcroft, John, 79
asymmetry, 51-52, 214
athletic activities, 100-114
augmentation surgeries, 65-66, 198-
    211, 216-219
Ayalah, Daphna, 90

B

Baby-Friendly Hospital Initiative, 122
Banks, Tyra, 199
Barbie, 53
bare breasts, 78-97
Barrymore, Drew, 91
basic knowledge, 2-6
bathing suits, 84, 85, 103-108, 111-112
benign illnesses, 177-180
Bierwagen, Karen, 31
Blue, Indigo, 94
body dysmorphic disorder (BDD),
    198-199
body image, 10-13, 46, 54, 62-68,
    74-76
boobiesexuals, 148
BRAC1/BRAC2 genes, 176
Brandon, Marja, 45
bras: buying tips, 32; care and
    maintenance, 41-42, 111; cup sizes,
    27, 31, 33-38; fitting guidelines,
    20-22, 30-42, 54-56, 74, 235-236;
    historical background, 22-25;
    marketing and manufacturing,

26-29, 40-41; maternity/nursing
    bras, 131; mature breasts, 228-230;
    measurement methods, 35-38;
    media images, 12-13; personal
    boob journal, 237; sizing chart,
    36-37; sports bras, 101, 103, 109-113;
    training bras, 13, 54-55
Brassiere, Phillip de, 24
Brava Breast Enhancement and
    Shaping System, 156
breast awareness activities, 16-17
breast-conserving surgery, 188
breastfeeding, 9, 80-83, 116-133, 159
breast lifts, 211
Breast of Canada calendar, 90
breast self-exams: basic care, 57, 153,
    171, 218; early cancer detection,
    165-167; procedures, 238-241
breast size and shape: basic
    knowledge, 8-9; breast
    enhancements, 57-58, 65-66, 156,
    199-200; cancer, 145-146; common
    concerns, 49-52; cosmetic surgeries,
    196-219; mature breasts, 222-231;
    media images, 11, 62-64; sexuality,
    144-146; size trends, 13; stereotypes,
    60-61; See also bras; reconstructive
    surgery
Breasts Not Bombs, 89
Brumberg, Joan Jacobs, 44
burlesque theater, 93-95
bustiers, 28

C

Cadolle, Herminie, 24, 28
cancer: basic knowledge, 180-185;
    benefit programs, 172; breast size
    and shape, 145-146; cancer-causing
    ingredients, 154; clinical trials, 172;

Acknowledgments

The roots of this book can be traced back to author Waverly Fitzgerald and media maven Whitney Keyes, in whose classroom I discovered my bliss. Nick O'Connell of The Writer's Workshop gently nurtured my novice writing attempts and pushed me to pursue my bigger book idea. Lilly Ghahremani of Full Circle Literary put her faith in a three-minute pitch at a writer's conference and devoted her time and energy to securing my publisher, Seal Press. My editor, Brooke Warner, worked diligently to refine my ideas into a coherent, logical, and readable manuscript.

This book reflects the different ways women perceive their breasts. I am grateful to those who sat down with me to share their personal breast stories and to others who anonymously answered my questionnaire or submitted their own mammoirs on my website. Their views and experiences shaped the direction of my research. Many other men and women recommended additional books, websites, and products to include.

Others instrumental in supporting my boobs along the way were, Jeri Rice both for her professional counsel and personal friendship; Kevin Winslow, the "udder man"; Meghan Arnette and the artists at Live Girls, who gave the stage to The Boob Lady; Marja Brandon and the teachers and students at Seattle Girls' School, who launched my educational presentations; and breast activists Dr. Paul Rapaport, Sue Richards, and Kathy Kiefer, who inspired me with their efforts to continue the boob dialogue.

Many thanks to the experts who granted interview requests and answered numerous phone and email inquiries: Dr. Robert Grenley, Dr. Drew Welk, Dr. Lisa Sowder, Dr. Edward Pechter, Dr. Richard Baxter, Dr. Brandith Irwin, Dr. John Sundsten, Judy Herrigel, Marcella Fleming Reed, Kate Starbird, and the extraordinary Amelia Ross-Gilson a.k.a. Miss Indigo Blue, the Twirly Girl. I am indebted to the staff at Seattle Cancer Care Alliance, including Tracy Cothran, Dr. Constance Lehman, and Dr. Julie Gralow. Thanks and gratitude to medical researcher Constantine Kaniklidis for sharing his vast knowledge of breast cancer with me and for encouraging me to look at all sides of a very complicated subject.

No book on breasts could be complete without the advice of those who dress them best. Special thanks to Victoria Roberts of Zovo Lingerie, Karen Bierwagen of Le Mystere, Jodi Gallaer of Jodi Gallaer Lingerie, Poupie Cadolle from House of Cadolle, Anne Dimond of Bella Materna, and Rebecca Apsan of La Petite Coquette.

Thanks also to Joni Morishita, artist, designer, and business partner, for her loyal and steadfast friendship and her early encouragement and faith in my abilities.

This book would not exist without the guidance and support of two women I met at the start of my journey: Amy Frazier, writer, teacher, and performer, and Jennifer Gerstenberger, writer, poet, and Urban Pixie. They generously offered their time and talents and stood by me every step of the way. Together we formed an impenetrable six-tit triangle of power filled with love, light, and laughter. I am blessed to have had them touch my life in such a remarkable way.

My family welcomed The Boob Lady with open arms and never questioned my choice of subject matter. My children, Will, Mayre, and James, expressed confidence in my success from the beginning, and each encouraged me in their own special way. My husband, Randy Squires, picked up the slack during my absence by cooking, driving carpool, and performing mundane household chores. He sat patiently and listened to my incessant boob banter, always assuring me that the topic held his interest. Even when I was frozen by fear or other insecurities, his faith in me never wavered. Randy has given me many gifts over the course of our twenty-five years together, including three wonderful children. It is this most recent offering—his love and encouragement to be my true and authentic self—for which I am eternally grateful.

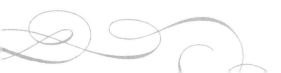

DUE DATE: 09-07-13
BARCODE: 33029062997424
TITLE: Boobs : a guide to your girls

DUE DATE: 09-07-13
BARCODE: 33029096012240

TITLE: Tantric sex for busy couples : ho

Item(s) checked out to p2664737.

#206 08-17-2013 5:02PM

About the Author

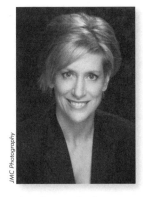

JMC Photography

Elisabeth Squires, a.k.a. The Boob Lady™, has been breast obsessed since her early teens. Her website, www.booksonboobs.com, is part of *BUST* magazine's Girl Wide Web and provides women with an essential forum to talk and learn more about their breasts. Squires, an internationally recognized breast expert, has worked with nonprofit organizations as a consultant, public speaker, grant writer, and volunteer fundraiser for the past twenty-five years. The daughter of a breast cancer survivor, she recently underwent surgery for a breast lift. She is the mother of three children, including a teenage girl. She lives with her family in Seattle.